Learning Disabilities - Neurological Bases, Clinical Features and Strategies of Intervention

Edited by Sandro Misciagna

Published in London, United Kingdom

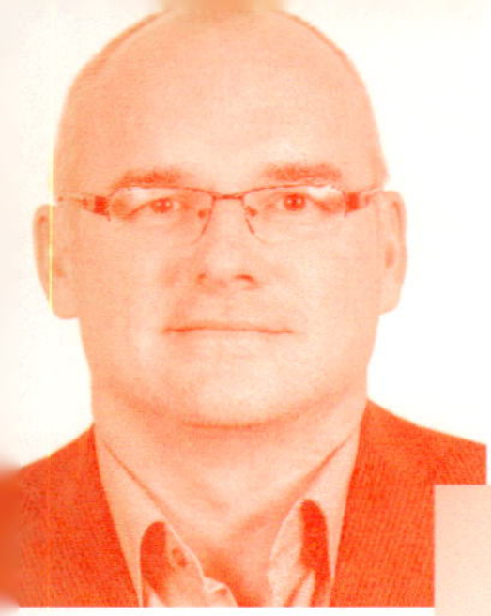
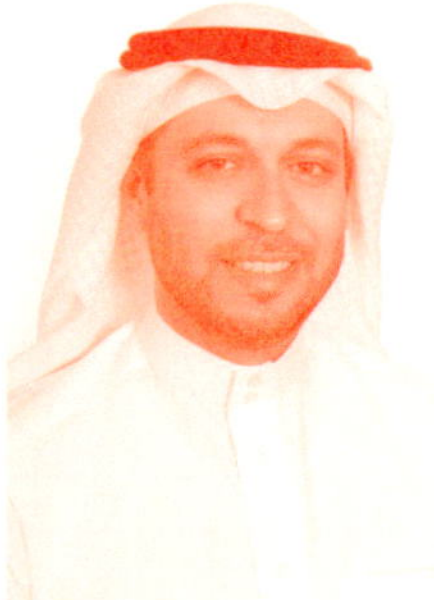
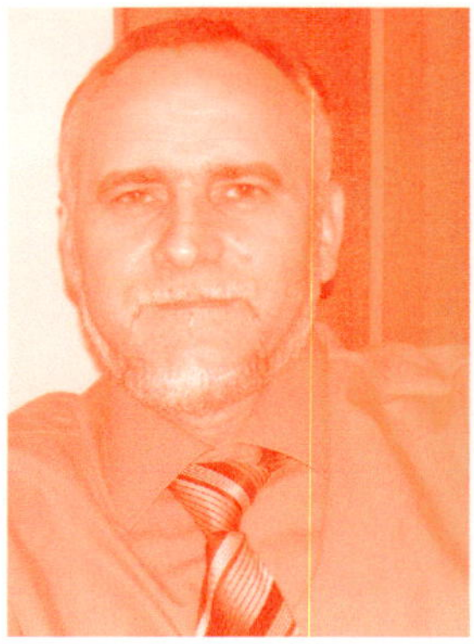
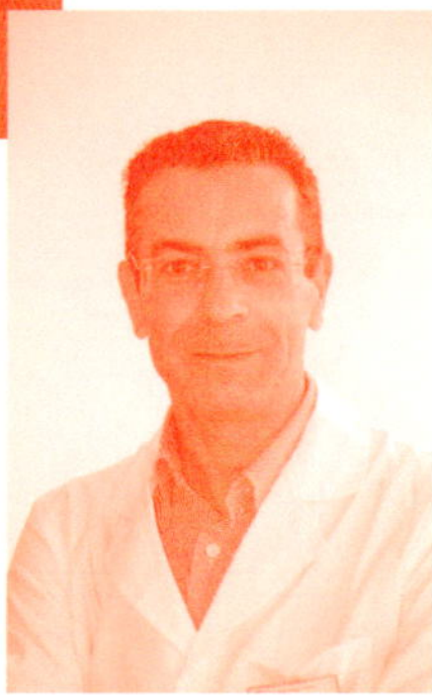
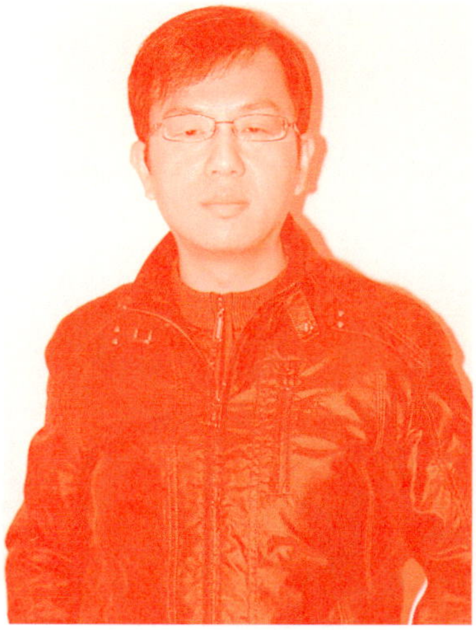
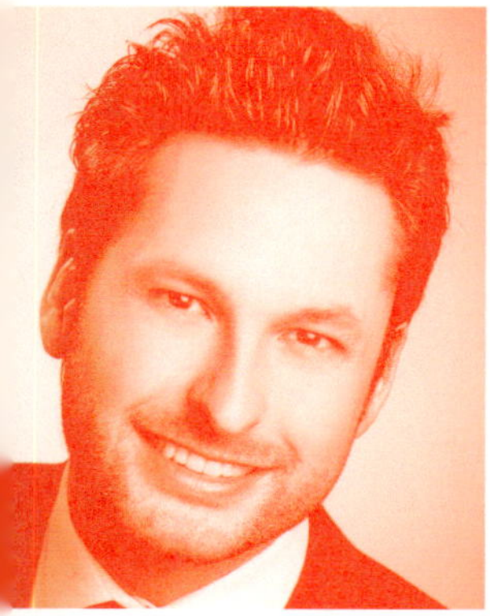
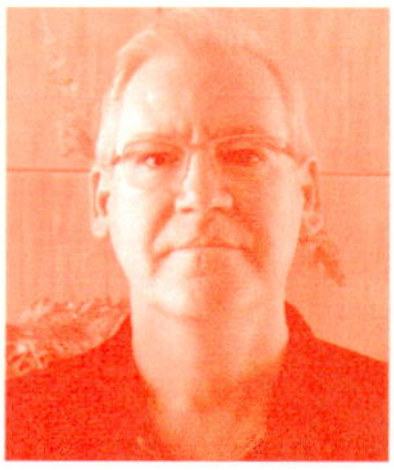

IntechOpen

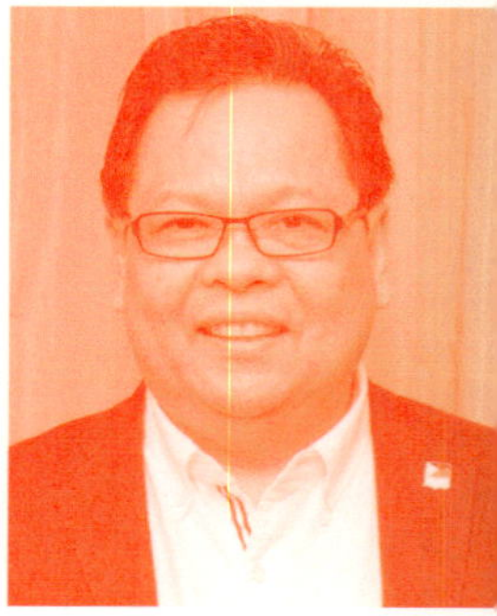
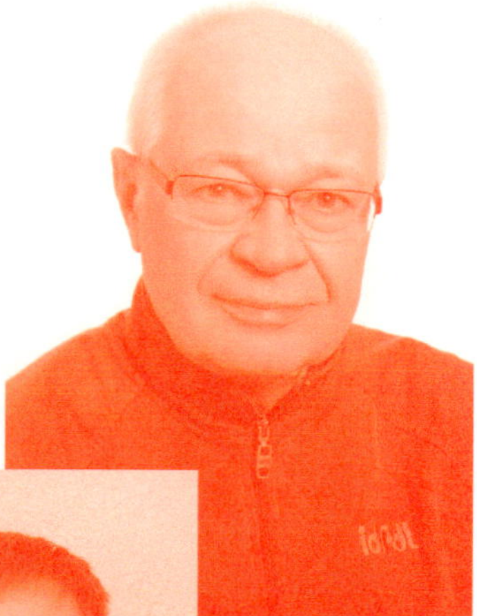
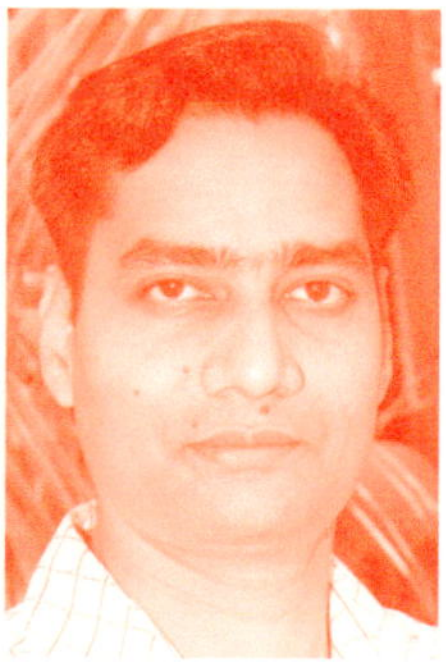
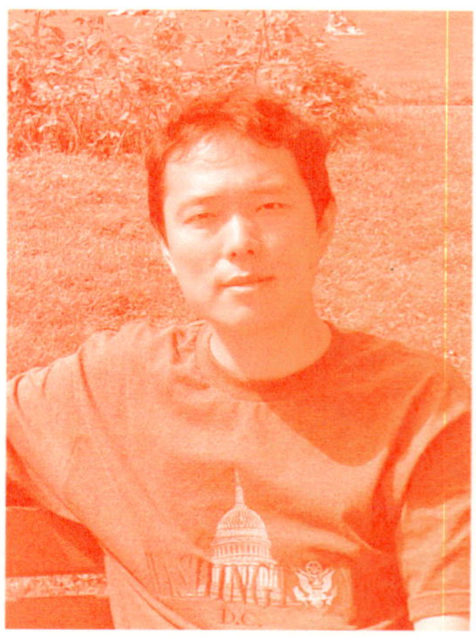
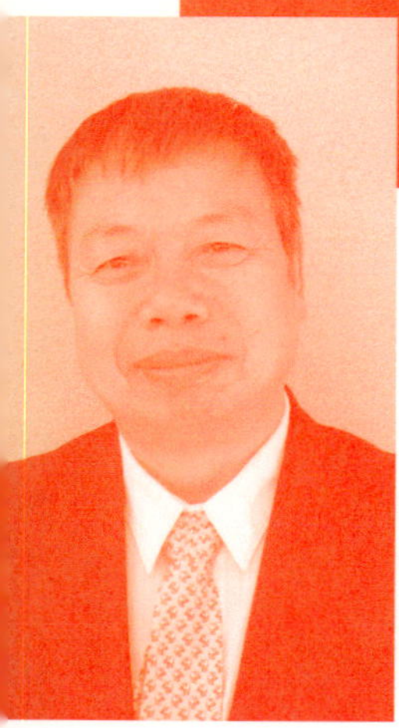
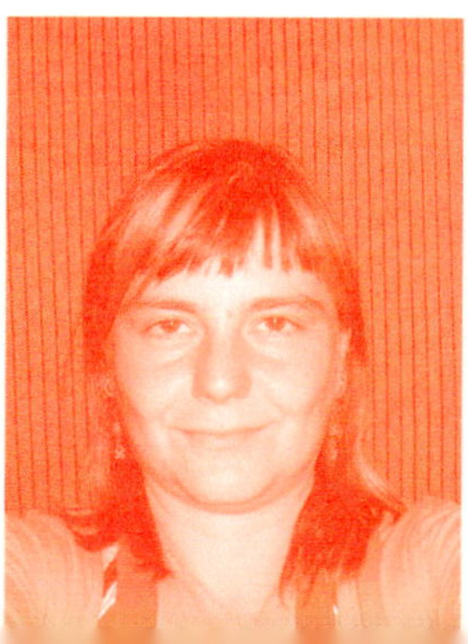

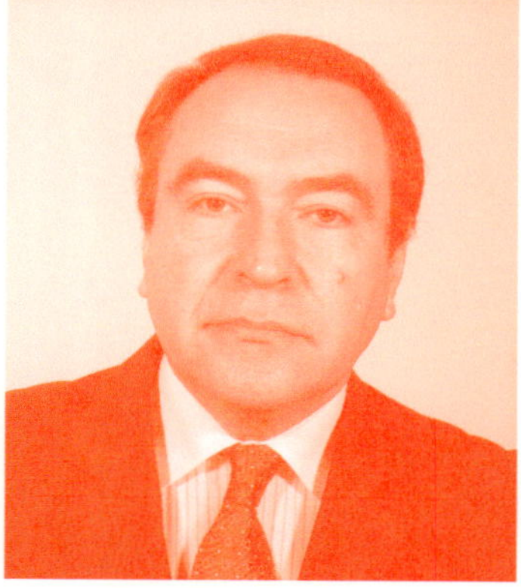

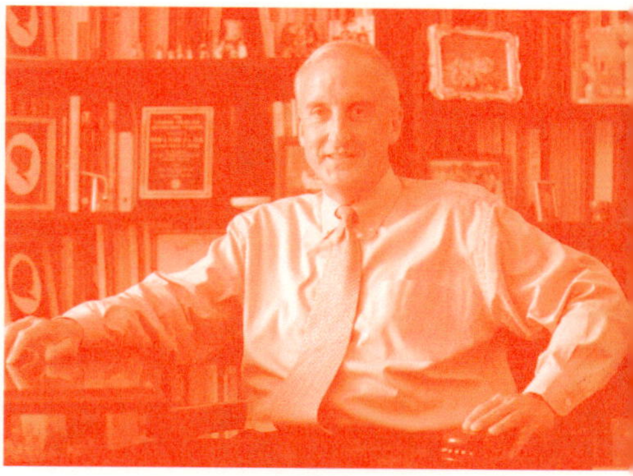

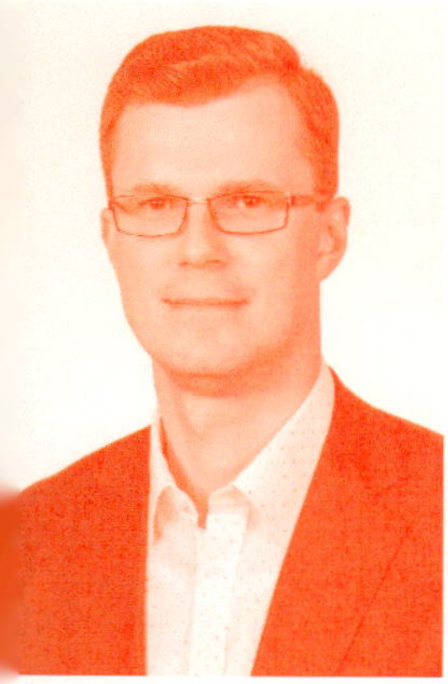

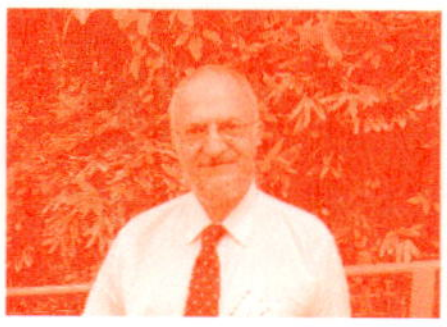

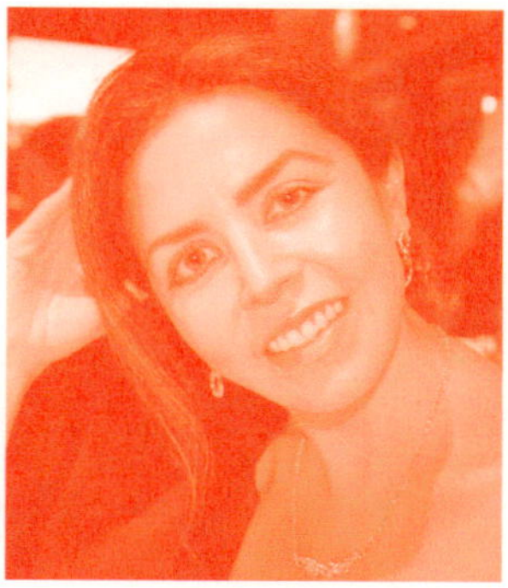

Supporting open minds since 2005

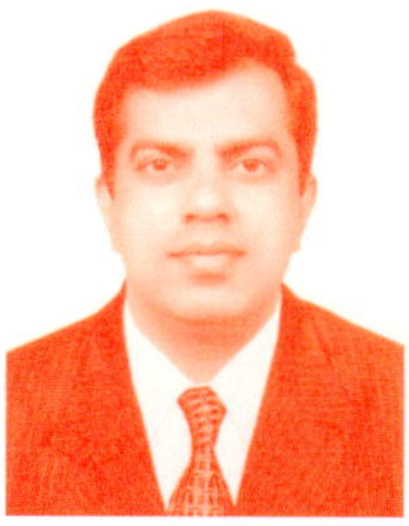

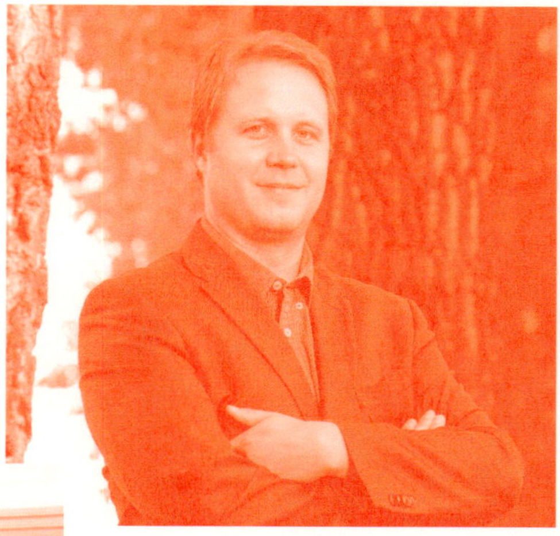

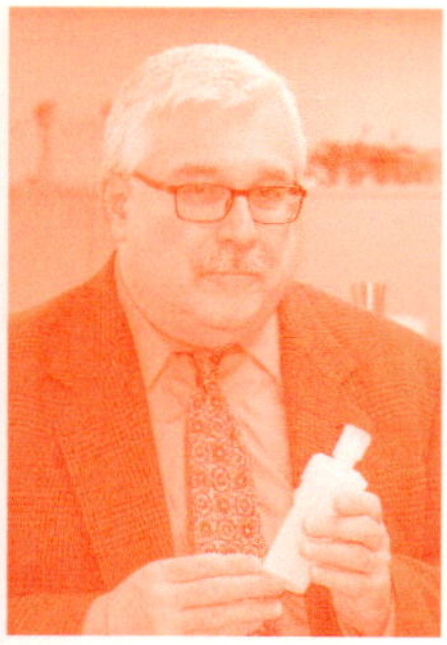

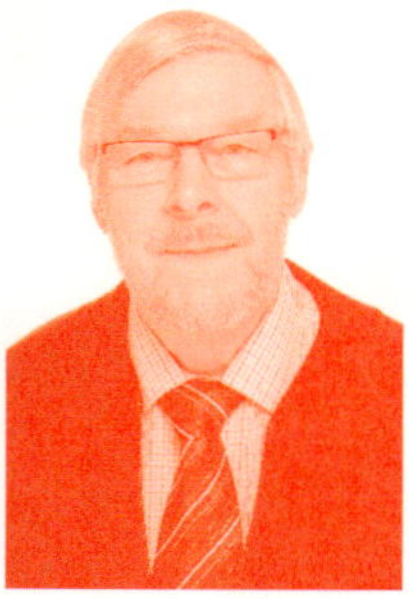

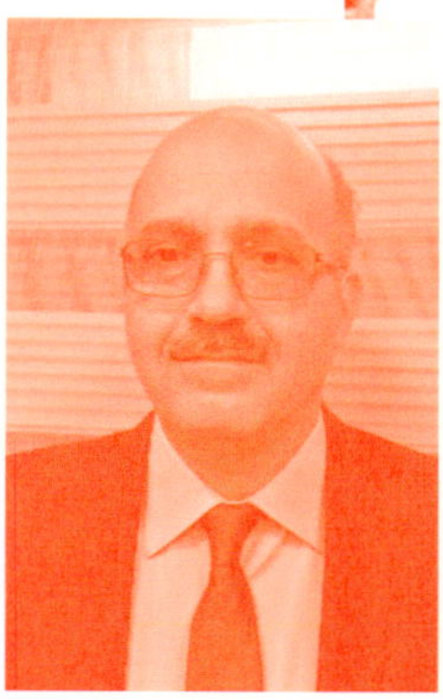

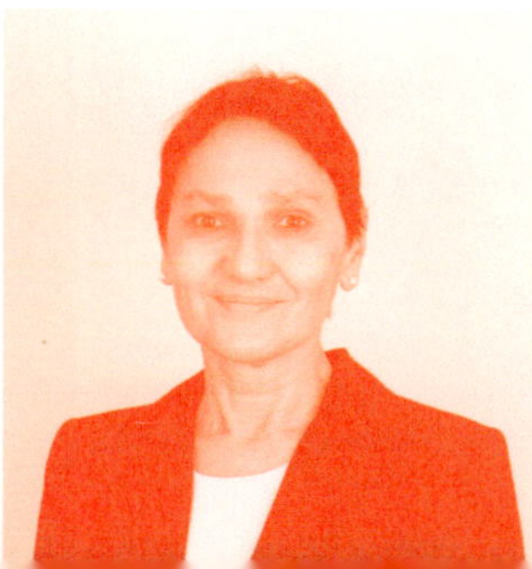

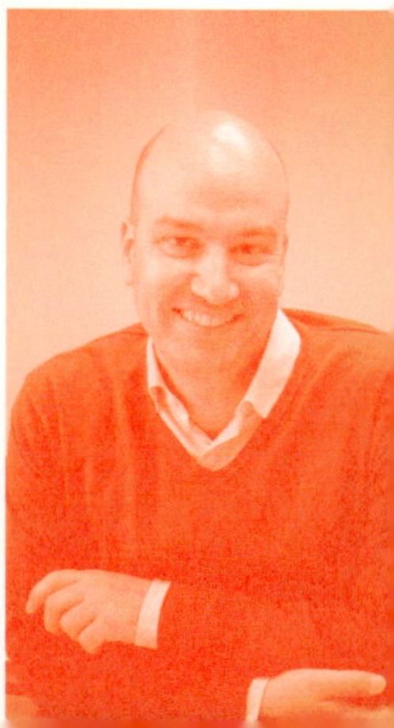

Learning Disabilities - Neurological Bases, Clinical Features and Strategies of Intervention
http://dx.doi.org/10.5772/intechopen.86684
Edited by Sandro Misciagna

Contributors
Işık Görker, Trisno Ikhwanudin, Suprih Widodo, Edgardo Domitilo Gerardo Morales, Ricardo Moura, Ingrid Ya I Sun, Ana Carolina Martins Cortez, Fernanda Dreux Miranda Fernandes, Rakgadi Grace Malapela, Gloria Thupayagale-Tshweneagae, Sandro Misciagna, Tatiana Volodarovna Tumanova, Tatiana Borisovna Filicheva, Diane Montgomery, Maria Tzouriadou, Maria Rontou, Connie Suk-Han Ho, Edmond Hong-Kei Cheung, Jocelyn Ching-Yan Kwok, Nada Pop-Jordanova

First published in London, United Kingdom, 2020 by IntechOpen
IntechOpen is the global imprint of INTECHOPEN LIMITED, registered in England and Wales, registration number: 11086078, 7th floor, 10 Lower Thames Street, London, EC3R 6AF, United Kingdom
Printed in Croatia

British Library Cataloguing-in-Publication Data
A catalogue record for this book is available from the British Library

Additional hard and PDF copies can be obtained from orders@intechopen.com

Learning Disabilities - Neurological Bases, Clinical Features and Strategies of Intervention
Edited by Sandro Misciagna
p. cm.
Print ISBN 978-1-83880-838-9
Online ISBN 978-1-83880-839-6
eBook (PDF) ISBN 978-1-83880-840-2

For EU product safety concerns:
IN TECH d.o.o., Prolaz Marije Krucifikse Kozulić 3, 51000 Rijeka, Croatia, info@intechopen.com or visit our website at intechopen.com.

Meet the editor

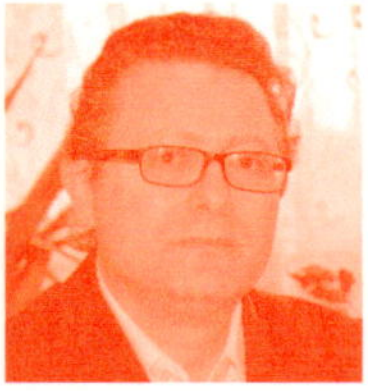

Dr. Sandro Misciagna was born in 1969. He received a degree in medicine in 1995 and in neurology in 1999 from Catholic University, Rome. From 1993 to 1995 he worked at a research laboratory studying cerebellar functions of mice; from 1994 to 2003 he studied cognitive and behavioural disorders; and from 2001 to 2003 he taught neuropsychology, neurology, and cognitive rehabilitation. In 2003 he obtained a PhD in Neuroscience with a thesis on the behavioural and cognitive profile of frontotemporal dementia. As a clinician, he has worked in neurological, neuro-rehabilitative, and neuropsychiatric clinics. Since November 2016 he has worked in the neurological department of Belcolle Hospital, Viterbo. His interests include epilepsy and neurophysiology.

Contents

Preface

Learning disabilities (LDs) consist of impairment in one or more cognitive domains such as written or spoken expression, reading, math, information processing, and memory. Individuals with LDs have lower than expected measured intelligence for their age. LDs negatively affect children, their families, and ultimately society. It is important to note that there is not a universal consensus regarding the definition of LDs.

According to the United States Office of Education (1977), the term "specific learning disability" means a disorder in one or more basic psychological processes involved in understanding or in using language, spoken or written, which may manifest itself in an imperfect ability to listen, speak, read, write, spell, or do mathematical calculations. The term includes such conditions as perceptual handicaps, brain injury, minimal brain dysfunction, dyslexia, and developmental aphasia. Such terms do not include children who have LDs that are primarily the result of visual, hearing, or motor handicaps, of intellectual disability, of emotional disturbance, or of environmental, cultural, or economic disadvantage.

According to the National Joint Committee on Learning Disabilities (1997), "learning disabilities" is a general term that refers to a heterogeneous group of disorders manifested by significant difficulties in the acquisition and use of listening, speaking, reading, writing, reasoning, or mathematical skills.

The Individuals with Disabilities Education Act (IDEA, 2004) defines "specific learning disability" as an impairment in one or more of the following cognitive domains: understanding or using written or spoken language, math, information processing, memory, or reading, including dyslexia, orthographic impairment (inability to memorize words), and hyperlexia (comprehension difficulties). The IDEA also includes in the definition of LDs conditions such as developmental aphasia, perceptual disabilities, brain injury, and minimal brain dysfunction.

Finally, the American Psychiatric Association (2013) defines "learning disorders" as specific disorders of reading, writing expression, or mathematics skills that are lower than expected for the individual's age, measured intelligence, and age-appropriate education level.

LDs affect approximately 10 percent of children in the United States. Of these children, about 40 percent have learning disabilities in language, reading, math information processing, or memory.

Language or speech impairment affects about 18.5 percent of American children. Dyslexia is the most common disability, affecting about 80 percent. Children with intellectual disability (7.4 percent) also have comorbidity with learning and emotional disturbances.

Other cognitive deficits, such as memory problems, attentional deficits, and difficulty managing social interactions are not typically considered LDs.

LDs are also common in children with attention deficit hyperactivity disorder (ADHD), chronic health conditions, or other mental and psychological disorders such as anxiety, depression, bipolar disorder, and obsessive compulsive disorder.

Risk factors for LDs include prenatal alcohol exposure, prematurity, low birth weight, early life malnutrition, and under-stimulating environment. Other risk factors include a family history of LDs such as dyslexia, ADHD, memory difficulty, and dropping out of school. Medical conditions associated with LDs include some neurological conditions (epilepsy or epileptic disorders, neurofibromatosis, tuberous sclerosis, complex Tourette syndrome), chromosomal disorders (Turner syndrome, Klinefelter syndrome, fragile X syndrome), certain chronic medical conditions (pediatric HIV infection, adolescent diabetes mellitus), and history of central system infection, irradiation, or traumatic brain injury.

Pathogenesis of LDs is not known. The full expression of LDs probably occurs as a result of intrinsic neuropathological factors (brain functions) in conjunction with environmental factors that include home factors (exposure to learn at home, degree of support provided in the home) and school factors (student–teacher interactions, level of stimulation provided by learning materials, classroom setting).

The most common LDs are dyslexia, writing disorders, and math learning disorder.

Reading disability (dyslexia) is in general the most frequent LD and is estimated to occur in approximately 5 to 12 percent of school-age children, depending upon the criteria used for definition. It consists in specific reading disorder such as difficulty identifying which letter/letter combination correlates with a particular sound (phonics and decoding), difficulty reading printed text smoothly and efficiently (reading fluency), and difficulty understanding what was read (reading comprehension).

Writing disability is estimated to occur in approximately 7 to 15 percent of school-age children. Writing disability consists of a range of disabilities including problems in composing sentences and text (excessive grammar and punctuation errors), difficulty with handwriting (copying efficiently from the chalkboard), difficulty with spelling (phonics, encoding), and problems properly organizing written text.

Math learning disorder is estimated to occur in 3 to 6 percent or 6 to 13.8 percent of children. Math learning disorder includes difficulty with mental representation of quantity (number sense) and difficulty in performing math calculations accurately (adding, subtracting, multiplying, dividing). Students with math LDs can also have difficulty with the language of math (difficulty correctly reading and understanding math symbols), word problems in math (correctly reading and understanding numbers and arithmetic symbols), and visuospatial organization of math problems.

LDs usually do not exist in isolation but co-occur with other learning cognitive and behavioral conditions. For example, among children with writing disability, 15 percent have coexisting reading and math disability, 14 percent have coexisting reading disability, and 13 percent have coexisting math disability.

It is difficult to accurately determine the frequency of co-occurrence of LDs with psychiatric conditions. However, most studies suggest LDs in 20 to 70 percent of children with behavioral or psychiatric conditions such as ADHD, anxiety, depression, or autism.

Differential diagnosis of LDs includes intellectual disability (formerly called mental retardation), psychiatric conditions (ADHD), sensorial deficits (hearing or vision impairment), sleep disorders, prenatal alcohol exposure (fetal alcohol spectrum disorders), genetic causes, neurological organic conditions (epileptic syndromes, progressive neurological disorders), or environmental factors.

Children with LDs must be submitted to an assessment to determine whether they are eligible for a treatment plan and the strategy of interventions.

Any assessment requires evaluation of speech, language, and mathematics by a qualified professional.

It is also useful to do a psychological and educational assessment that includes behavior and environment.

This book formulates a hypothesis to explain neurobiological bases of LDs, provides examples of LDs, and discusses assessment and treatment strategies. I hope it will contribute to preventing individuals from dropping out of school and enhancing life outcomes for those with LDs.

Sandro Misciagna, MD, PhD.
Belcolle Hospital,
Viterbo, Italy

Section 1

General Definition, Epidemiology and Neurobiological Bases of Learning Disabilities

Chapter 1

Concepts and Ambiguities in the Field of Learning Disabilities

Maria Tzouriadou

Abstract

Scholars and researchers have constantly argued due to the ambiguity and a lack of consensus in the scientific community in defining what constitutes a learning disability. The difficulty in identifying a universal term is reflected in the multiple terms that are used interchangeably (e.g. learning disabilities, specific learning disabilities, dyslexia, minimal brain dysfunction). Most commonly accepted and used definitions (e.g. IDEIA) can be considered ambiguous as it excludes certain conditions and describes characteristics in terms of abilities, processes, and achievement without discrimination between these terms. The only constant criterion (across definitions) is the discrepancy criterion that is the discrepancy between ability and achievement. In this context, it is important to note the differences in conceptualizing ability and academic achievement. Currently, the scientific community appears to agree that (a) learning disabilities are a distinct disability manifesting in students with low academic achievement, (b) it is a developmental disability that impacts individuals across their lifetime, and (c) it is a product of the interaction between genetic and environmental contributing factors, with environmental factors being determining by sociocultural conditions. Interventions addressing learning disabilities are not always evidence-based; interventions can be influenced by socioeconomic circumstances and policy decisions. Consequently, it is necessary to approach learning disabilities with a holistic and system-based approach rather than try to differentially diagnose them.

Keywords: learning disabilities, dyslexia, discrepancy criterion, evidence-based intervention RTI PSW

1. Introduction

Over the past years, learning disabilities (LD) or specific learning disabilities (SLD) have emerged as the most studied upon and renowned classification of special education with the term becoming synonymous with special education itself due to how frequently students are placed under this category. Nonetheless, it is also the special education category which has brought the most disagreement between scholars, researchers, and educators to this day, given that LD have not been established as a distinct discipline; that is, until now no causal relationship has been determined between the phenomenology of LD and the factors which cause them. Despite formal definitions, a lack of understanding of their nature and their interpretation exists, which indicates that the main goal of a distinct discipline is not fulfilled [1]. Without the understanding of their nature and interpretation, scientific standpoints regarding learning disabilities remain "into question" or "unfounded", and this constitutes the very root of the "identification problem" that is the lack of consensus on how to better define a classification category for LD [2]. Over a course of more than 100 years of studies, we have been unable to provide a unanimous and conclusive answer to a simple question: What are learning disabilities? Today, we believe that we know a lot about their characteristics and the implemented practices, but we have not yet answered the question whether they represent a distinct category of students with low academic achievement or they are a construct into which all low-performing students can be classified under. These two aspects have been meticulously studied over time, albeit not cohesively; consequently, even today some claim that LD represent a specific difficulty, since these children have high intelligence, while others believe that this category includes every child who is unable to learn. Since the beginning of the twenty-first century, scientists from various disciplines, but mostly educators, often come across parents' questions such as "My child, who goes to kindergarten, writes backwards, is this dyslexia?", "Will my child be a future Einstein?", "My child has trouble understanding meanings. Could this be dyslexia?", or "My child is distrait and performs poorly at school. Could he or she be having learning disabilities?" These scientists have attempted, through international organizations, such as the Learning Disabilities Association (LDA), to functionally operationalize the field—that is, to answer whether it is a scientific discipline with particular characteristics or a "pseudoscience", which covers all and nothing—and they have tried to identify the operational characteristics that would help children reach their full potential within the context of school and society.

2. Epistemological ambiguities of the field

Up until the 1960s, education had shown no interest in learning disabilities. Nevertheless, legislated compulsory education, the study of the school drop-out phenomenon, and the development of school's knowledge-based character have led to the creation of a new classification category, none other than LD. The fact that school success was associated with an individual's subsequent social and professional success contributed also to the creation of this distinct category given that LD pertained to individuals who had the potential of success due to their attributed higher cognitive skills. Over the course of time, this perception has consolidated, and learning disabilities have become the most important category of special education. An important indicator of this is the following: programs for children with LD congregate the highest number of students with special educational needs. 2.5 million of American school students approximately 5% from the total public school enrolment identified with learning disabilities in 2009. These students represented 42% of the 5.9 million school-age children. This percentage varies across states [3]. For example, in Kentucky, 3.18% of students belong in the specific learning disabilities category, while in Massachusetts and Port Island, the corresponding figures are 9% and 9.6% [3]. Similar differentiations are currently observed both in Canada and in certain European countries [4]. The variety of prevalence reflects various factors, like the diversity of the population belonging in this category; the increasing school pressure for higher achievement, which has led to higher standards; the different criteria used for the assessment of achievement; as well as the criteria applied to delineate the field of learning disabilities. The presence of such determining factors has resulted in LD student rates to fluctuate among US states. Consequently, LD represents the largest field within special education.

Across time, various definitions have been formulated, attempting to demonstrate the field's key characteristics. However, each one of them has been vague, figurative, negative instead of affirmative, and tautological or excessively broad or restrictive. Each subsequent definition attempted to correct the preceding ones. Therefore, their analysis is imperative, not with the objective of formulating a new definition but to broaden the description and notably the understanding of what learning disabilities actually are.

The term learning disabilities was coined by Kirk, who also devised their first definition [5]. This definition introduced for the first time the concept of disorders in the psychological processes involved in academic learning. Nevertheless, ambiguities in the field's delineation can still be found in this definition. For example, it mentions that disabilities refer to *retardation*, *disorder*, *or delay* but does not proceed to determine any difference between these terms. The definition also introduces the element of exclusion from other conditions of deficit, suggesting the case of differential diagnosis. Exclusion, however, is not a criterion for specifying the characteristics that differentiate LD from other conditions. Despite its ambiguities, Kirk's definition marked the establishment of the new field of LD and became the basis for every formal definition in the USA.

The acknowledgement of LD as an independent scientific field demanded the adoption of an operational definition, which would delineate its scope as a distinct category of special education. Such a definition was suggested by the US National Advisory Committee of Handicapped Children in 1968 [6]; it formed the basis for educational policies regarding children with LD and was included in the Individuals with Disabilities Education Act (IDEA) in 1997 [7]. Respectively, research in Europe and mainly in Britain focused on specific reading difficulties—dyslexia—and, even since the 1960s, there was the development of associations and treatment centers for children with this disorder [8, 9]. An important figure in the study of dyslexia in Britain was Critchley, who devised a definition for developmental dyslexia; according to his definition, it is a learning disorder which is initially manifested with difficulties in reading and later with "odd" spelling and difficulties in the use of written language. It is of cognitive nature and genetically determined. It is not caused by intellectual disability or lack of social and cultural chances, wrong instruction techniques, or emotional factors. Moreover, it is not due to any obvious structural cerebral insufficiency. Finally, Critchley did not agree with the use of the term "learning difficulties", because he believed that the children's only difficulty had to do with language [10]. Miles had another important scientific contribution in the study of dyslexia in Britain by conducting a large diachronic study during 1970–1980 on 14,000 children. According to the findings of this study, 3% of students showed severe symptoms of dyslexia and 6% mild symptoms. Miles also accepted that it was a hereditary disorder [11]. Rutter and his colleagues carried out epidemiological studies on children with reading difficulties and through them exhaustively highlighted specific reading difficulties. He argued that the terms and identification process used for dyslexia were chaotic and confusing, which is caused by the inability to interpret the nature of learning problems and may be confused with general reading retardation [12, 13]. In 1978, the British Department of Education and Science commissioned a committee to introduce a special education law in Britain, Wales, and Scotland in the spirit of normalisation and integration, a study that resulted in the Warnock Report (1978) which was adopted and became a law in 1983 [14]. In this law, it seems that an approach of low performance has been adopted under the term special educational needs regarding LD, with more than 18% of the student population being represented under this category. In this case dyslexia was not included as a category in special education, despite it being recognized as one. This is due to the fact that Britain adopted a purely pedagogical model at the administrative and practical level to address any educational needs of children. Most European countries have adopted Kirk's LD definition using the terms dyslexia or learning disabilities [4].

In the USA, on the other hand, studies on better understanding the nature of LD and determining best practices in their identification continued. In 1989, the National Joint Committee on Learning Disabilities, based on new evidence and scientific findings, attempted to eradicate inherent ambiguities in the identification of the field, by formulating the following definition:

Learning disabilities is a general term that refers to a heterogeneous group of disorders manifested by significant difficulties in the acquisition and use of listening, speaking, reading, writing, reasoning, or mathematical abilities. These disorders are intrinsic to the individual, presumed to be due to central nervous system dysfunction, and may occur across the life span. Problems in self-regulatory behaviors, social perception, and social interaction may exist with learning disabilities but do not by themselves constitute a learning disability. Although learning disabilities may occur concomitantly with other disabilities (e.g. sensory impairment, intellectual disabilities, emotional disturbance) or with extrinsic influences (such as cultural or linguistic differences, insufficient or inappropriate instruction), they are not the result of those conditions or influences [15]. Regarding this definition, Kavale et al. [16] highlights that the term "in general" is vague, much like the term "specific" in the IDEA's definition, thus allowing various interpretations.

In 2004, the IDEA regulation maintained the same definition of SLD as previous versions of the law and regulations. Notably, an attempt to expand the identification process occurred by including both a process based on the child's response to scientific, research-based intervention, such as response to intervention (RTI), and the use of other alternative research-based procedures, such as the Patterns of Strengths and Weakness (PSW) model. The IDEA definition, found in US Code (20 U.S.C. & 1401 [17]), reads as follows:

> *"The term 'specific learning disability' means a disorder in one or more of the basic psychological processes involved in understanding or in using language, spoken or written, which disorder may manifest itself in the imperfect ability to listen, think, speak, read, write, spell, or do mathematical calculations.*
>
> *Such term includes such conditions as perceptual disabilities, brain injury, minimal brain dysfunction, dyslexia, and developmental aphasia.*
>
> *Such term does not include a learning problem that is primarily the result of visual, hearing, or motor disabilities, of mental retardation, of emotional disturbance, or of environmental, cultural, or economic disadvantage" [18].*

This official definition introduces the "specific" aspect of the disorder for the first time, through the ambiguous distinction "in one or more", without specifying how many problems there could be in order for the disorder to be considered specific. Moreover, it provides no clarification of what specific means, if, for example, it refers to particular traits in the relevant subjects and the psychological structure or whether the term "specific" suggests that the disorder is idiopathic [19] that is of unknown cause. This definition also seems to introduce a hierarchy of processes, with language being dominant, whether oral or written. Furthermore, the disorder is not connected with difficulties in academic achievement alone but also with cognitive deficits (reasoning disorders), a trait that reflects what we nowadays call "metacognitive function". No mention of central nervous system dysfunctions appears yet, but there are references to similar cases deriving from neurological disorders.

Based on this legislation, educators are asked to identify if student suspected of SLD fails to show sufficient progress in achievement according to age-based and grade-level standards. This procedure provides important information and highlights a model of strengths and weaknesses in achievement and aptitudes. Intra-individual differences or variability are sometimes cited as an indication of SLD. The ability-achievement discrepancy is also taken into account as part of the process.

It is also argued that qualified staff should provide appropriate instruction. Students who have not received it cannot be considered as having SLD. Key instruction elements mainly regard reading, which, according to age, should be taught systematically:

- Phonemic awareness
- Phonics
- Vocabulary development
- Reading fluency, including oral reading skills
- Reading comprehension strategies

*Source: National Institute of Child Health and Human Development (NICHD) [20].

Schools also need to make frequent assessments of students' progress and inform parents. The gathered data might show the effectiveness of an instruction strategy or program. If the student does not exhibit any signs of progress, an extension may be granted—with the consent of the parents—which may not exceed 60 days.

Finally, the reauthorization regulations (NCLB) [21] included the statement that it is necessary to apply approaches to the instruction of reading that are supported by scientifically based reading research, mainly based on social construction. Concerning the instruction of reading, it has been argued that it may also be due to the over-representation of minorities in special education [22]. The reauthorized definition allowed US states to not use the IQ-achievement discrepancy or not provide intelligence tests as part of the diagnostic procedure and to include the RTI criterion as part of the diagnostic procedure.

The DSM uses the term "specific learning disorder". Revised in 2013, the current version, DSM-5, broadens the previous definition to reflect the latest scientific understanding of the condition.

The diagnosis requires persistent difficulties in reading, writing, arithmetic, or mathematical reasoning skills during formal years of schooling. Symptoms may include inaccurate or slow and effortful reading, poor written expression that lacks clarity, difficulties remembering number facts, or inaccurate mathematical reasoning. Current academic skills must be well below the average range of scores in culturally and linguistically appropriate tests of reading, writing, or mathematics. The individual's difficulties must not be better explained by developmental, neurological, sensory (vision or hearing), or motor disorders and must significantly interfere with academic achievement, occupational performance, or activities of daily living. Specific learning disorder is diagnosed through a clinical review of the individual's developmental, medical, educational, and family history, reports of test scores and teacher observations, and response to academic interventions [23].

There was intense research on an international level—but mostly in the USA—and millions of dollars were spent in the pursuit of the field's delineation [24]. However, as of yet there is no crystallized description of the condition but rather a generalized depiction of a group of school children with difficulties in learning. We may know a lot about the condition, but we do not know why LD exist.

Even the definitions' points of convergence do not lead to a uniform interpretation of their nature. For this reason, in numerous studies and research, SLD are approached from different perspectives, and different terms are used to describe them, such as learning disabilities, specific learning disabilities, dyslexia, specific language impairment, attention deficit hyperactivity disorder, etc. But in all formal definitions, the element of ability-achievement discrepancy appears constantly.

The problem of discrepancy raises a reasonable question: "What is the meaning of concepts such as intelligence or general cognitive ability, learning or cognitive processes, and academic achievement—concepts that are included in every definition of SLD—and what is the causal relationship between them?" [4]. Unless this question is resolved, the identification of the field will remain vague and contentious. Since conceptual and scientific definitions did not facilitate the identification of the SLD field, an operational description of the condition was required for practical implementation. The phenomenon of intra-individual differences was first studied, particularly the possibility of some "malfunctioning" of certain abilities in contrast to the normal development of others. These developmental imbalances could become apparent in discrepancies of intelligence functions, which are included in intelligence testing, such as the Wechsler Intelligence Scale for Children (WISC). WISC composites can be used to identify profiles of strengths and weaknesses, which can distinguish students with SLD from other groups of students with average or low overall intelligence function scores. This analysis method of developmental discrepancies led to controversy regarding the nature of SLD. Is the profile of these students unique among this entire population? Does the profile of SLD subtests significantly differ from other cases with normal intelligence quotients? [25].

In a meta-analysis of studies, Kavale and Forness [17] could not determine a specific WISC-based profile for students with LD, because, despite the imbalances among the subtests or between the verbal and practical part of the criterion, the differences were deemed statistically insignificant. Thus, they argued that "specific" profiles could only be indicative of the children's competencies and incompetencies, an element useful in the planning of pedagogical treatment. Studies with similar results also came to the same conclusion [26]. Failure to identify intra-individual discrepancies of cognitive abilities reinforced the notion that discrepancies could be identified between intelligence and performance indices, a feature that is first introduced in the field's delineation by Bateman's definition [27].

Gradually, this criterion of ability and achievement has become a dominant feature in the identification of SLD. The main problem with this approach was that, while the WISC test remained the constant criterion for the intelligence quotient (IQ), achievement was being assessed with various formal and informal criteria. For this reason, the discrepancy criterion was disputed [28]. A further reason of doubt was that meta-analyses of studies determined a change in the rate of students with LD when different criteria were applied. For example, analyses of findings in the state of Colorado showed that 26% of students did not meet the criterion, while 30% only did so in reading and maths. By applying a different criterion for achievement among the same sample, 5% of students met the criterion in maths and 27% in reading [28]. In another meta-analysis of findings, Cone, Wilson, and Bradley found that, in the state of Iowa, 75% met the discrepancy criterion [29]. In a similar study, Kavale and Reese [30] noted discrepancy rates between 33% and 75% depending on the tests being used. Thus, Lyon et al. came to the conclusion that discrepancy as a primary criterion of determining LD is more harmful than beneficial for children, because achievement criteria involve various external factors, such as the educator, the infrastructure, the curriculum, etc.; these factors can neither be isolated nor interpret the complex interactions between "deficit" and pedagogical/social factors, which need to be taken into consideration during the diagnostic procedure [31].

About 50 years ago, Cruickshank described a vague picture of students with LD as students who are classified differently in each state [32]. The lack of definition of the nature of LD and the ambiguity regarding the causal relationships between learning abilities and academic achievement, but also the question of whether they represent a specific disorder and what that means, led to overgeneralisations of the term, with all children with difficulties in academic achievement to be thought of presenting LD or, on the contrary, to sub-generalizations of the term based on one symptom, which appears in most cases of LD, usually in reading difficulties. It is a fact that 90% of students with LD exhibit reading difficulties [30]. But is this problem primary or secondary? Which cases of reading difficulties might fall within the range of LD? According to studies, children with reading difficulties of various causes are impossible to be distinguished from children who fall within the category of SLD (dyslexia), as stipulated in IDEA's definition [33, 34]. But even in cases of specific reading difficulties, namely, dyslexia, it has been argued that students with this disorder find themselves at the lowest point of the normal distribution of reading ability [35]. Ysseldyke et al., in their study of students who were diagnosed as having LD and students who were not diagnosed but were at the lowest level of the reading ability distribution, found no psychometric differences in the performance of the two groups [36]. Based on these results as well as other studies, Algozzine concluded that in general, LD as a category is "non-existent and useless" [33]. Also, the fact that the majority of these children exhibit reading difficulties has led—mainly in Europe—to the equation of LD with dyslexia, which, while representing one of their symptoms, according to IDEA's definition, has ended up becoming an autonomous scientific field. Thus, mainly in Europe, LD have been equated with dyslexia on the basis of the unclear criteria of low reading performance and the exclusionary elements included in all LD definitions.

The lack of consensus has led to the development of two trends on an international professional and administrative level. On the one side stand, those who accept SLD as a distinct group [37–40] and, on the other, those who relate them to every student of low academic achievement [41]. In most countries, though, educators apply solely the criterion of excluding low intelligence quotients; that is, they aim to differentiate between students who have an intellectual ability and associated adaptive skill deficits and those who have SLD [42].

In summary, it seems obvious that lack of consensus among scholars, researchers, and practitioners regarding the key elements which distinguish the LD category from other low-achievement categories, as well as the lack of common understanding of their nature and causes, has led the field to stagnation. Two contradictory positions in the general debate exist. One identifies disabilities with the innate-specific learning inadequacies of these students, while the other considers them an "umbrella" category, which covers a wide range of students with low achievement without developmental specificities. For those supporting the "umbrella" characterization, LD is a construct of the modern educational system, which, according to Senf [38], has tried to purify general education like a sociological sponge, which is most "absorbing" when academic demands are rigid or the parents' pressure for achievement is higher. This sponge also absorbs not only the individual differences of students but also a variety of pedagogical, behavioral, and psychosocial problems, which can impede school learning. However, with no scientific delineation of the field, LD cannot represent a scientific entity.

3. Contemporary frameworks to identify LD

For this reason, researchers today try to redefine the field of SLD in order to answer the question whether SLD constitute a scientific category or they represent one of the groups with lower achievement, not in need of a special treatment or specially designed instruction. As recently argued [43, 44], the field delineation should summarize all the pre-existing knowledge reflected in the various definitions and the applied pedagogical practices; this will help identify the degree of the deficiency's contribution as well as the contribution of influences by a variety of exogenous factors.

In the USA, educational reform efforts have placed emphasis on the application of evidence-based instructional approaches with the aim of improving the instruction of reading, which has been the focus of research both in the USA and internationally for over 30 years. A major concern that emerged from research was the failure of educational systems to close the gap between children, particularly those with disabilities and those belonging to minorities [45].

Despite the redefinitions and educational regulations, there are still ambiguities and contradictions regarding the conceptualisation and identification of LD. Although there have been attempts to determine why they exist, and many neurobiological researchers have tried to attribute them to disorders of the central nervous system (CNS), so far their causes have not been established [18, 46]. The identification framework of intelligence-achievement discrepancy is still used internationally by those who view LD as a distinct disorder, while the low-achievement model is applied by those who talk of a non-distinct group of low achieving students.

In the USA, school districts in various states have started supplementing the traditional model of testing (e.g. intelligence-achievement discrepancy) with RTI. As aforementioned RTI is considered a viable method for identifying students with LD. In a national survey, 72% of teachers and 54% of parents were in favor of this decision, mainly because RTI's approach facilitates early intervention and pre-referral services [47]. This way, inappropriate referrals to special education are reduced, and at the same time preventative intervention model is created for students who otherwise been referred for special education services after they demonstrated school failure. In recent years, another framework—the pattern of strengths and weaknesses (PSW)—has emerged with the tendency to prevail; although not covered by federal law regulations, it is widely accepted and used in the USA because it supports research-based practices [40, 48].

Thus, depending on the theoretical approaches toward LD, today there are four framework models that can be used for the conceptualisation and identification of SLD, especially in the USA [41]. Proponents of the non-distinctive nature of the disorder have adopted the *low-achievement framework*, which does not take into account the element of unexpected underachievement. Proponents of the distinctive nature of the disorder use one or more of the three remaining frameworks: *intelligence-achievement discrepancy*, *response to instruction-intervention*, and *intra-individual differences* (PSW) [49]. A key element to the disorder's distinctive character is the concept of unexpected underachievement; this is presented by children which should be able to learn but cannot demonstrate scholastic success, without the existence of other learning obstacles, and while receiving adequate instruction. Therefore, the key aspect in assessing the identification's validity is to determine which of the frameworks produce a unique group of low achievers [31]. A valid classification should reflect measurements that provide functionality to the construct of unexpected underachievement [50].

The traditional framework of intelligence-achievement discrepancy (IAD) remains dominant in the identification both in the USA and internationally, despite the controversy it has provoked. It is a determining method of identifying students with SLD when they present significant discrepancy between cognitive ability, as typically measured by IQ, and academic achievement, as measured by standardized reading, writing, and mathematical tests [51]. This framework has been criticized for its reliability both in terms of aptitude tests and achievement tests, due to the multidimensional nature of LD and the errors in psychometric measurements.

Response to intervention (RTI) is another framework which, as mentioned, facilitates instruction both in general education and specific interventions for students who do not meet the core curriculum level. In order for a student to be considered at risk for academic difficulties, the student's assessments are compiled, and his or her progress is monitored after specific interventions. Following the implementation of interventions, when there is still discrepancy in achievement and growth, then the student is considered to have LD [52]. This model is used in the USA, while another similar pedagogical model of dynamic assessment is used in Britain. This framework has also received criticism, on the grounds that the use of multiple assessments in class to identify students with lower achievement in each subject is an unstable method, always depending on the group comprising the class. With the use of either a single test or the scores in multiple tests, it is hard to notice the latent of a student's abilities and determine the cut-point that would place him or her in the LD group.

As it has been said that the framework of the pattern of strengths and weaknesses is allowed under the provision of alternative research-based practices in the IDEA. There are different PSW models, like the concordance-disconcordance model [44], the dual discrepancy/consistency model (also referred to as cross-battery assessment; [40]), and the discrepancy/consistency model [48]. These three models differ in methodology, but they converge on the fact that students can be identified as having SLD when they demonstrate unexpected academic underachievement and corresponding weakness in one or more specific cognitive abilities related to the area of the academic deficit [53]. However, in practice, students can be often identified with SDL through demonstration of a pattern of strengths and weaknesses only in academic achievement domains [49]. Moreover, multiple individual differences might be present, which accumulate the errors of measurements and render them unreliable.

In a recent survey regarding the frameworks being used by school psychologists in the USA, Cottrell and Barrett [54], looking at a sample of 471 school psychologists, found out that 63.1% were almost always using the intelligence-achievement discrepancy (IAD) framework. 49.3% were using the RTI framework in most cases, and 29.4% were using the PSW framework in almost every case. However, they could not determine which framework was being primarily employed. For instance, 31.5% reported that they had been using the RTI framework most of the times, while only 17.8% reported that they were using this framework exclusively. In order to find out which one is being primarily employed, Maki and Adams surveyed 461 school psychologists in 2017 [55]. They discovered that only 30.4% reported primarily using the IAD framework, while they were primarily using almost equally the RTI (34.5%) and the PSW (35.1%) framework, respectively.

Benson et al. [56], in another national-level US-based survey with 1317 school psychologists, found out that 37% were using IAD, even in states where it is not included in the diagnostic procedure. Fifty-one percent were using RTI [56]. Finally, approximately 53% reported that they were using PSW. In the same survey, 49.2% reported that they were participating in academic screening procedures, which include monitoring of early literacy, oral reading fluency, reading comprehension, early numeracy, math computation, math concepts and applications, spelling, and written expression prompts, according to the age of the students. Many of the participants reported a combined use of RTI and PSW, RTI and IAD, and PSW and IAD. This last survey confirms the lack of consensus regarding identification procedures among professionals in the identification of SLD.

4. Conclusions

In order to summarize the international research effort, it seems that scientists concur that LD represent a distinct group of students with low academic achievement, regardless of the terms used to describe them (dyslexia, learning difficulties, special learning difficulties, special reading difficulties, etc.). They also agree that it is a matter of developmental disorder with implications across the life span. As a developmental problem, LD follow a course from the beginning of life and are determined by the interaction of innate factors with the environment, much like development itself. LD do not comprise a distinguishable entity like other developmental phenomena but a combination of traits; their common element is the existence of discrepancies in cognitive function and achievement, and they appear to be incompatible with social and cultural demands and expectations. The source of their heterogeneity is not exclusively biological or environmental but rather a product of synergy between biological and social processes, which promote development and contribute to the formation of these functional systems. It may never be possible to find a dividing line or a criterion that distinguishes students with SLD from those with an overall low performance. The controversy between scientists may carry on. Decisions are not always based on scientific but mainly social, economic, and political reasons. It is widely accepted that the root of LD is a disorder that already exists within the child; however, it is the child's interaction with the world around him or her that shapes how this disorder manifests. Such a systemic perspective demands an exhaustive understanding and an interdisciplinary approach. A lot remains unresolved before we can answer the questions regarding the nature and interpretation of LD. We know a lot from empirical data, but we are not in the position to complete the puzzle and provide an answer to the main question which has to do with the field's identification. Until then, we must continue to assess and fully understand the developmental path of each child and to take into account all the factors involved in the development of learning disabilities.

Author details

Maria Tzouriadou
School of Early Childhood Education, Aristotle University of Thessaloniki, Thessaloniki, Greece

*Address all correspondence to: tzour@nured.auth.gr

References

[1] Cattell RB. The time taken up by cerebral operations. Mind. 1886;**11**: 220-242, 377-392, 524-538

[2] Doris J. Defining learning disabilities: A history of the search for consensus. In: Lyon GR, Gray DB, Kavanagh JF, editors. Better Understanding Learning Disabilities. Baltimore: Brooks; 1993. pp. 97-116

[3] National Center for Learning Disabilities (NCLD). Learning Disability Fast Facts. 2011. Available from: www.ld.org/ld-basics/ld-explained/basic-facts/ld-fast-facts

[4] Tzouriadou M. Learning Disabilities: Issues of Identification and Identification. Prometheus: Thessaloniki; 2011

[5] Kirk SA. Educating Exceptional Children. Boston: Houghton Mifflin; 1962

[6] National Advisory Committee on Handicapped Children (NACHC). Special Education for Handicapped Children (First Annual Report). Washington, DC: Department of Health, Education, and Welfare; 1968

[7] Individuals with Disability Education Act Amendments of 1997 [IDEA]. 1997. Available from: https://www.congress.gov/105/plaws/publ17/PLAW-105publ17.pdf

[8] Arkell H. The Edith Norrie Letter Case. London: Helen Arkell Centre; 1973

[9] Wepman JM, Cruickshank WM, Deutsch CP, Morency AS, Strother GR. Learning disabilities. In: Hobbs N, editor. Issues in the Classification of Children. Vol. 1. San Francisco: Jossey-Bass; 1975. pp. 300-317

[10] The CM, Child D, Naidoo S. Specific Dyslexia: The Research Report of the ICAA Word Blind Centre for Dyslexic Children. London: Pitman; 1972

[11] Miles TR. Understanding Dyslexia. London: Hodder and Stoughtn; 1978

[12] Rutter M. The concept of dyslexia. In: Wolffand H, MacKeith R, editors. Planning for Better Learning. London: Heinemann; 1969. p. 129

[13] Rutter M, Tizard J, Whitmore K, editors. Education, Health and Behaviour. London: Longman Green; 1970

[14] Report W. Special Educational Needs. Report of the Committee of Enquiry into the Education of Handicapped Children and Young People. London: Her Majesty's Stationery Office; 1978

[15] National Joint Committee on Learning Disabilities. Letter from NJCLD to Member Organizations. Topic: Modifications to the NJCLD Definition of Learning Disabilities; 1989

[16] Kavale KA, Spaulding LS, Beam AP. A time to define: Making the specific learning disability definition prescribe specific learning disability. Learning Disability Quarterly. 2009;**1**:39-48. DOI: 10.2307/25474661

[17] Kavale KA, Forness SR. A meta-analysis of the validity of Wechler scale profiles and recategorizations: Patterns of parodies? Learning Disabilities Quarterly. 1984;7:136-156. DOI: 10.2307/1510314

[18] Individuals with Disabilities Education Improvement Act [IDEIA]. Pub. L. No. 108-446, 118 Stat. 2647. 2004

[19] Eisenberg L. Definitions of dyslexia: Their consequences for research and policy. In: Benton AL, Pearl D,

editors. Dyslexia: An Appraisal of Current Knowledge. New York: Oxford University Press; 1978

[20] National Institute of Child Health and Human Development. Report of the National Reading Panel: Teaching Children to Read: An Evidence-based Assessment of the Scientific Research Literature on Reading and Its Implications for Reading Instruction: Reports of the Subgroups (NIH Publication No. 00-4754). Washington, DC: U.S. Government Printing Office; 2000

[21] US. Department of Education. No Child Left Behind. 2004. Available from: http://www.ed.gov/nclb/landing.jhtml

[22] Donovan MS, Cross CT. Minority Students in Special and Gifted Education. Washington, DC: National Academy Press; 2002. Available from: http://www.nap.edu/catalog/10128.html

[23] American Psychiatric Association. Diagnostic and Statistical Manual of Mental Disorders. 5th ed. Arlington, VA: American Psychiatric Association; 2013

[24] Hallahan DP, Mercer CD. Learning Disabilities: Historical Perspectives. Washington, DC: US Department of Education, Office of Special Education Programs; 2001

[25] Kaufman AS. The WISC-R and learning disabilities assessment: State of the art. Journal of Learning Disabilities. 1981;**14**:520-526

[26] Naglieri JA. Factor structure of the WISC-R for children identified as learning disabled. Psychological Reports. 1981;**49**:891-895. DOI: 10.2466/pr0.1981.49.3.891

[27] Bateman B. An educator's view of a diagnostic approach to learning disorders. In: Hellmuth J, editor. Learning Disorders. Vol. 1. Seattle: Special Child Publication; 1965. pp. 219-239

[28] Shepard LA, Smith ML, Vojir CP. Characteristics of pupils identified as learning disabled. American Educational Research Journal. 1983;**20**:309-331. DOI: 10.3102/00028312020003309

[29] Cone TE, Wilson LR, Bradley CM, Reese JH. Characteristics of LD students in Iowa: An empirical investigation. Learning Disability Quarterly. 1985;**8**:211-220

[30] Kavale KA, Reese JH. The character of learning disabilities: An Iowa profile. Learning Disability Quarterly. 1992;**15**:74-94. DOI: 10.2307/1511010

[31] Lyon GR, Shaywitz JM, Shaywitz BA, Torgesen JK, Wood FB, Schulte A, et al. Rethinking learning disabilities. In: Finn CE, Rotherham AJ, Hokanson C Jr, editors. Rethinking Special Education for a New Century. Washington DC: Thomas B. Fordham Foundation and Progressive Policy Institute; 2001. pp. 259-287

[32] Cruickshank WM. The Brain-Injured Child in Home, School, and Community. Syracuse, NY: Syracuse University Press; 1967

[33] Algozzine B. Low achiever differentiation: Where's the beef? Article Commentary. 1985;**52**:72-75. DOI: 10.1177/001440298505200109

[34] Fletcher JM, Shaywitz SE, Shankweiler DP, Katz L, Liberman IY, Stuebing KK, et al. Cognitive profiles of reading disability: Comparisons of discrepancy and low achievement definitions. Journal of Educational Psychology. 1994;**86**:6-23

[35] Shaywitz SE, Fletcher JM, Hallahan JM, Schneider AE, Marchione KE, Stuebing KK, et al. Persistence of dyslexia: The Connecticut

longitudinal study at adolescence. Pediatrics. 1999;**104**:1351-1359

[36] Ysseldyke JE, Algozzine B, Shinn MR, McGue M. Similarities and differences between low achievers and students classified learning disabled. Journal of Special Educatio. 1982;**16**:73-85

[37] Kirk SA. Illinois test of psycholinguistic abilities: Its origin and implication. In: Hellmut J, editor. Learning Disorders. Seattle: Special Child Publications; 1968

[38] Senf GM. LD research in sociological and scientific perspective. In: Torgesen JK, Wong BYL, editors. Psychological and Educational Perspectives on Learning Disabilities. New York: Academic Press; 1986. pp. 27-53

[39] Naglieri J, Bornstein B. Intelligence and achievement: Just how correlated are they? Journal of Psychoeducational Assessment. 2003;**21**:244-260. DOI: 10.1177/073428290302100302

[40] Flanagan DP, Alfonso VC, Sy MC, Mascolo JT, McDonough EM, Ortiz SO. Dual discrepancy/consistency operational definition of SLD: Integrating multiple data sources and multiple data-gathering methods. In: Alfonso VC, Flanagan DP, editors. Essentials of Specific Learning Disability Identification. Hoboken, NJ: Wiley; 2018. pp. 329-430

[41] Hallahan DP, Pullen PC, Ward D. A brief history of the field of learning disabilities. In: Swanson H, Harris KR, Graham S, editors. Handbook of Learning Disabilities. New York, NY: The Guilford Press; 2013. pp. 15-32

[42] Fletcher JM, Coulter WA, Reschly DJ, Vaughn S. Alternative approaches to the definition and identification of learning disabilities: Some questions and answers. Annals of Dyslexia. 2004;**54**:304-331

[43] Waber DP. Rethinking Learning Disabilities: Understanding Children Who Struggle in School. New York: Guilford Press; 2010

[44] Hale JB, Alfonso V, Berninger B, Bracken B, Christo C, Clark E, et al. Critical issues in response-to-intervention, comprehensive evaluation, and specific learning disabilities identification and intervention: An expert white paper consensus. Learning Disability Quarterly. 2010;**33**(3):223-236

[45] Lemons CJ, Fuchs D, Gilbert GK, Fuchs LS. Evidence-based practices in a changing world: Reconsidering the counterfactual in education research. Educational Researcher. 2014;**43**:242-252. DOI: 10.3102/0013189X14539189

[46] American Psychiatric Association. Diagnostic and Statistical Manual of Mental Disorders—Text Revision. 4th ed. Washington, DC: Author; 2000

[47] National Center for Learning Disabilities (NCLD). Early Help for Struggling Learners: A National Survey of Parents and Educators. Author; 2002. Available from: http://www.ld.org/press/PR2003/survey_findings.pdf

[48] Naglieri JA, Feifer SG. Pattern of strengths and weaknesses made easy: The discrepancy/consistency method. In: Alfonso VC, Flanagan DP, editors. Essentials of Specific Learning Disability Identification. Hoboken, NJ: Wiley; 2018. pp. 431-474

[49] Fletcher JM, Miciak J. The Identification of Specific Learning Disabilities: A Summary of Research on Best Practices. Texas Center for Learning Disabilities: Houston University of Houston; 2019

[50] Stuebing KK, Fletcher JM, LeDoux JM. Validity of IQ-discrepancy classifications of reading disabilities: A meta-analysis. American Educational

Research Journal. 2002;**39**(2):469-518. DOI: 10.3102/00028312039002469

[51] Fletcher JM, Lyon GR, Fuchs LS, Barnes MA. Learning Disabilities: From Identification to Intervention. 2nd ed. New York, NY: Guilford Press; 2019

[52] Kovaleski J, VanDerHeyden AM, Shapiro ES. The RTI Approach to Evaluating Learning Disabilities. New York, NY: Guilford Press; 2013

[53] Alston-Abel NL, Berninger VW. Relationships between home literacy practices and school achievement: Implications for consultation and home–school collaboration. Journal of Educational and Psychological Consultation: The Official Journal of the Association for Educational and Psychological Consultants. 2017;**28**(2):164-189. DOI: 10.1080/10474412.2017.1323222

[54] Cottrell JM, Barrett CA. Defining the undefinable: Operationalization of methods to identify specific learning disabilities among practicing school psychologists. Psychology in the Schools. 2016;**53**(2):143-157

[55] Maki KE, Adams SR. A current landscape of specific learning disability identification: Training, practices, and implications. Psychology in the Schools. 2018;**56**:18-31. DOI: 10.1002/pits .22179

[56] Benson NF, Maki KE, Floyd RG, Eckert TL, Kranzler JH, Fefer SA. A national survey of school psychologists' practices identifying specific learning disabilities. School Psychology (Washington, D.C.). 2019;**4**:1-12. DOI: 10.1037/spq0000344

Chapter 2

The Prevalence and Gender Differences in Specific Learning Disorder

Işık Görker

Abstract

Learning process including reading, writing, and arithmetic skills in children requires a normal cognitive development period. The presence of signs of disabilities of these skills needs clinical assessment of a specific learning disorder (SLD), a neurodevelopmental disorder. Specific learning disorder which is defined in DSM-V with three types has various prevalence rates according to age, sex, developmental process, environmental factors, and different assessments applied in studies. Comorbidity with other mental disorders reveals more severe symptoms of it. And also if clinical and educational interventions are not performed, behavioral and emotional symptoms may accompany this diagnosis. In this chapter, studies on the prevalence of specific learning disorder are reviewed by considering these factors.

Keywords: specific learning disorder, dyslexia, dyscalculia, prevalence, child

1. Introduction

Specific learning disorder (SLD) is defined as a neurodevelopmental disorder that includes the difficulties in understanding or learning, problems in writing or written expression, and difficulties in the perception/calculation of the numbers. These problems make the academic performance of the child lower than expected. This disorder is originated from biology affecting the acquisition or perception capabilities of the brain for the verbal and nonverbal information processes. There is an abnormality of cognitive level associated with behavioral findings in its etiology [1]. Therefore, it is defined as a failure to meet approved grade-level standards in listening comprehension, reading comprehension, basic reading and reading fluency skills, written expression, mathematics calculation, and/or mathematics problem-solving, despite age-appropriate learning opportunities and instruction [2]. These deficits are persistent and significantly interfere with academic achievement, occupational performance, or activities of daily life [3].

SLD is a multifactorial disorder which has in its etiology a genetic predisposition and family load, developmental and cognitive factors, language spoken, and environmental factors including the level of education and socioeconomic situation. In many studies, gender, level of intelligence, higher family history of learning disabilities, low parental education, the exposure during pregnancy to the use of medicines, exposure to radiation, smoking, infections, hypoxia, complicated deliveries, hypoxia during labor, premature labor, low birth weight, low Apgar score, neonatal jaundice, convulsions, developmental delay, low-income families, and low socioeconomic status, leading to the occurrence of the SLD, are defined as predeterminants [4–11]. In the clinical examination of SLD, children's developmental, medical, educational, and family history are assessed. Test scores and teacher observations and response to academic interventions are also evaluated. For SLD, current academic skills must be well below the average range of expected scores given the person's chronological age (e.g., at least 1.5 standard deviations (SD)) below the population mean for age and age-appropriate education in culturally and linguistically appropriate tests of reading, writing, and/or mathematics [2, 3, 12] with normal levels of intelligence functioning (considering an intellectual coefficient (IQ) score greater than 70) [1]. These problems cannot be explained with mental retardation, loss of sense (vision or hearing), other psychiatric or neurological disorder, psychosocial difficulties, insufficiency of the language to be used in the academic environment, or education problems. The types like reading disorder (dyslexia), written expression disorder (dysgraphia), and mathematics disorder (dyscalculia) can be seen together or separately.

SLD are usually apparent in the early years of school; some children can show great learning difficulties later on, enabling diagnosis to be made at any point after formal education starts and in adolescence and even adulthood [1]. If treatment approaches are not initiated at an early age, the lives of children and adolescents with SLD are adversely affected due to academic failure. In almost 40% of cases dropout of school. Due to low academic failure, lack of self-confidence, social and behavioral problems may cause emotional problems. This can lead to anxiety disorders, depressive symptoms, somatic complaints, adaptation problems, and difficulties in maintaining a permanent job in the future [1, 13–16].

2. The prevalence rates evaluated in studies of specific learning disorder

The number of the prevalence studies with diagnostic criteria or scales for SLD is low. On the other hand, SLD is accepted as relatively frequent and is not known sufficiently [17–19]. There have been many studies on SLD from the past to today, and different ratios have been announced on the prevalence. The frequency and prevalence of the SLD are stated in various reports with different rates depending on the size of the sample and the inclusion criteria. For example, Al-Yagon et al. reported different prevalence rates that included 1.2% from Greek epidemiologic study in 2004 and 20.0% from a study in Australia in 2000 [20]. A lifelong prevalence estimative of learning disability was found to be 9.7% in children from 3 to 17 years of age by the 2003 National Survey of Children's Health (NSCH) in the USA [4]. The study in Finland in 2001 reported a prevalence of 21.2% in school-aged children referred to special education [15]. Del'Homme et al. reported this prevalence of 28.0% in 2004 [21]. In an epidemiological study with 2174 primary school children in Turkey by using checklists, the probable prevalence rates were found to be 13.6% [7]. An important problem that is making the performance of the epidemiological studies harder is the lack of generally accepted definitions or diagnostic criteria for SLD and evaluations based only on a scale or other assessments that measure the level of academic achievement. DSM-V located the diagnosis of SLD into the category of neurodevelopmental disorders and included severity ratings for its assessment. This means that SLD is conceptualized as a dimensional developmental disorder that occurred as a result of multiple risk factors interacting with each other. One of the important changes is the elimination of IQ-achievement discrepancy criterion in DSM-V despite the exclusion criterion of intellectual disability. IQ-discrepancy criterion was taken into consideration in DSM-IV criteria, so prevalence rates have found different in studies. For example, in one of the recent studies with 1633 German children in third and fourth grades, the SLD frequency was investigated according to DSM-V criteria, and three different findings were calculated according to the 1, 1.25, and 1.5 standard deviations. Accordingly, the reading disorder for children having 1 as the standard deviation was estimated at 6.49%, written expression disorder was 6.67%, and mathematics disorder was 4.84%; the reading disorder for children having 1.25 as the standard deviation was estimated to be 5.14%, written expression disorder was 6.86%, and mathematics disorder was 3.31%; the reading disorder for children having 1.5 as the standard deviation had an estimated value of 3.8%, written expression disorder was 5.02%, and mathematics disorder was 2.39% [3]. In another study with 1618 Brazilian children and adolescents from second to sixth grades, different prevalence rates were found of SLD by using DSM-IV and DSM-V criteria. These rates were 7.6% for SLD (global) impairment, 5.4% for writing, 6.0% for arithmetic, and 7.5% for reading impairment. The prevalence rates were found to be higher by using DSM-V criteria as they expected [22]. In DSM-V, the American Psychiatric Association reports that the SLD prevalence of children from different languages and cultures is 5–15%, the prevalence of reading disorder is 4–9%, and the prevalence of mathematics disorder is 3–7 [1].

When the reading, writing, and mathematics difficulties were separated, or when reading and mathematics difficulties were grouped together, in studies conducted in different countries, the difficulty rates were found to be different from each other. In previous studies, researchers have suggested that arithmetic and reading functions may depend on similar cognitive predictors [23–25]. It was found that the same phonological processing abilities that are considered to influence growth in reading also appear to contribute to growth in general computation skills [24]. And it was determined that there is a relationship between deficits in processing words and accessing arithmetic facts in long-term memory by Geary [23]. Arithmetical skill is a skill that is based on counting, which involves number words and the use of phonological skills. Because counting involves the activation of number words, the association in long-term memory between problem and answer could be represented, at least in part, in the same phonetic and semantic memory systems that support word recognition. Therefore, it was suggested that the co-occurrence of reading and arithmetic disabilities might reflect a more general deficit in the representation or retrieval of information from semantic memory [26]. The roles of family history and genetic load are considered in reading difficulties and mathematics difficulties, and it is suggested that phonologic problems stated in the etiology of the reading difficulties can create different rates of reading difficulties interculturally, depending on the spoken language. The difficulties in phonemic compliance led to phonologic problems leading to reading difficulties; so, it is suggested that reading difficulties are seen less in countries that have good phoneme-grapheme harmony, and there are higher rates in countries that have poor phoneme-grapheme harmony. Majority of the studies suggested that the prevalence of reading disorder was 5–17% [27]. In the study conducted with 1476 children in 1983, the mathematics disorder rate was 3.6%, and the reading disorder was 2.2% [28]; in the study conducted by Lewis et al. [29] in 1994 with 1056 children who were 9–10 years old, the mathematics disorder was found to be 1.3%, and the reading disorder was 3.9%. In the study conducted by Miles et al. [30] in 1998, the reading disorder prevalence was suggested to be 4.19%, and also in the study of Badian [31] in 1999 with 1075 children, the reading disorder was suggested to be 6%, and the mathematics disorder was suggested to be 3.9%. The studies of Badian [31] and Lewis et al. [29] were designed to obtain an estimation of the prevalence of combined reading and arithmetic, reading only, and arithmetic-only disabilities. Badian found that the prevalence rate in arithmetic and reading was 3.4%, for reading only 6.6%, and for arithmetic only 2.3%. And Lewis reported prevalence proportions as follows: 2.3% for combined reading and arithmetic, 3.9% for reading only, and 1.3% for arithmetic only. When different methods and materials are used in the prevalence studies, different results are obtained as in the studies of Badian and Lewis. While Badian evaluated comprehension in reading, Lewis evaluated word weakness. Although they are both reading processes, they in part require different cognitive skills. Therefore it leads to the identification of a different population of weak readers. Furthermore, another source of variable results across studies is the use of different cutoff scores for the identification of reading and arithmetic disabilities as in these studies. Similarly Dirks et al. [32] found a higher percentage of combined reading and arithmetic disabilities than the disability in reading or arithmetic alone by using different assessments as in studies of Badian and Lewis et al. And they emphasized that children with combined reading and arithmetic disabilities were different from those who had reading or arithmetic disability alone in terms of cognitive and neuropsychological differences [32].

In 2007, Von Aster et al. [33] performed a study with 337 children, and the reading disorder was found in 3.3%, writing disorder in 5.7%, and mathematics disorder in 1.8%. In the study conducted by Landerl and Moll [34] in 2010 with 2586 children, the reading disorder was found to be prevalent in 2.9%, written expression disorder was 4.1%, and mathematics disorder was 3.2%. A study in France detected prevalence rates of dyslexia between 5.0 and 10.0% in school-age children in the same year [35]. Dhanda and Jagawat [36] worked with 1156 children, and the reading disorder was 22%, written expression disorder was 22%, and mathematics disorder was 16%. After the findings with different results according to the different standard deviations in 2014 by Moll et al. [3], Cappa et al. [37] performed a study in 2015 that reading disorder was found to be 4.75%; Fortes et al., on the other hand, found the cases of prevalence of SLD to be 7.6%, with reading disorder at 7.5%, writing disorder at 5.4%, and mathematics disorder at 6.0% [22]; Gorker et al. determined 3.6% for reading, 6.9% for writing, and 6.5% for mathematics difficulties [7].

The roles of family history and genetic load are considered in reading difficulties and mathematics difficulties, and it is suggested that phonologic problems stated in the etiology of the reading difficulties can create different rates of reading difficulties interculturally, depending on the spoken language. The difficulties in phonemic compliance led to phonologic problems leading to reading difficulties; so, it is suggested that reading difficulties are seen less in countries that have good phoneme-grapheme harmony, and there are higher rates in countries that have poor phoneme-grapheme harmony [27]. For instance, according to the UK Parliamentary Office of Science and Technology, the prevalence of SLD reading disorder in the UK is higher due to differences in pronunciation of a letter in English than most languages and inconsistencies in writing and vocabulary [38].

There are no prevalence studies of mathematic disability that considered longitudinal data, except with 210 sample that were followed multiple times during a 4-year period that found 9.6% by Mazzocco and Myers (2003) [39]. Although large cohort studies do exist with a larger sample initially, a small subset of children is identified as potentially displaying mathematics difficulties, so these studies have not provided a detailed comparison of the cognitive and demographic characteristics of subtypes of learning difficulty. And also two studies investigated the prevalence of specific learning difficulties in arithmetic skills but did not assess their types (e.g., number sense, number facts, and mathematical reasoning) [3, 22]. Different levels of prevalence results of mathematics disability are attributed to some methodological differences of studies. One of them is the method that uses IQ-achievement discrepancy. In retrospective population-based study with 5718

	Specific learning disorder (%)	Reading disorder (%)	Written expression disorder (%)	Mathematic disorder (%)	Reading + mathematics disorder (%)	Methodology
Badian [28]		2.2		3.6		Questionnaire
Lewis et al. [29]		3.9		1.3	2.3	Standardized tests
Gross-Tsur et al. [45]				6.55		Standardized tests
Miles et al. [30]		4.19				Questionnaire and standardized tests
Badian [31]		6		3.9	3.4	Standardized tests
	20					Questionnaire
Hein et al. [42]				6.6		Standardized tests
Ramaa and Gowramma [46]				5.54–5.98		Standardized tests
Mazzocco and Myers [39]				9.6		Standardized tests
Desoete et al. [43]				2.27–6.59		Standardized tests
Barbaresi et al. [40]				5.9–13.8		Questionnaire and standardized tests
Altarac et al. [4]	9.7					Questionnaire
Von Aster et al. [33]		3.3	5.7	1.8		Standardized tests
Barahmand [41]				3.76		Standardized tests
Lagae [27]		5–17				Standardized tests
Dirks et al. [32]		19.9		10.3	7.6	Standardized tests
Landerl and Moll [34]		2.9	4.1	3.2		Questionnaire and standardized tests
Geary [44]				5.4		Standardized tests
Taanila et al. [15]	21.2					Questionnaire

	Specific learning disorder (%)	Reading disorder (%)	Written expression disorder (%)	Mathematic disorder (%)	Reading + mathematics disorder (%)	Methodology
Dhanda and Jagawat [36]		22	22	16		Questionnaire
Al-Yagon et al. [20]	1.2					Questionnaire
Moll et al. [3]		6.49	6.67	4.84		DSM-V criteria 1 standard deviation
		5.14	6.86	3.31		DSM-V criteria 1.25 standard deviation
		3.8	5.02	2.39		DSM-V criteria 1.5 standard deviation
Cappa et al. [37]		4.75				Questionnaire
Fortes et al. [22]	7.6	7.5	5.4	6		DSM-V criteria checklists and questionnaire
Gorker et al. [7]	13.6	3.6	6.9	6.5		Checklists
Morsanyi et al. [8]		5.6		6		DSM-V criteria and standardized tests

Table 1.
Overview of the prevalence rates of specific learning disorder, reading disorder, written expression disorder, mathematics disorder, and reading-mathematics disorder.

children assessed prevalence rates based on different formules and found 5.9% to 13.8% and also significantly more frequent among boys than girls [40]. Barahmand studied 1171 children who are at grades 2–5 and found 3.76% [41]. Others defined mathematics disability by the severity of the mathematics impairment have used performance cutoffs on standardized tests. Some of these studies and their prevalence rates are as follows: 3.6 and 3.9% by Badian's studies [28, 31], 1.3% by study of Lewis et al. [29], 6.6% by study of Hein et al. [42], 9.6% by studies of Mazzocco and Myers [39], 5.9–13.8% by study of Barbaresi et al. [40], 2.27–6.59% by study of Desoete et al. [43], 5.6–10.3% by study of Dirks et al. [32], and 5.4% by study of Geary [44]. The other researchers defined mathematics disability using a 2-year achievement delay as a diagnostic criterion. They found the prevalence rates to be 6.55 [45] and 5.54–5.98% [46]. Recently, Devine et al. compared mathematics and reading difficulties with 1004 primary school children and reported that there were no differences between boys and girls when a discrepancy criterion was applied [47]. The study in 2018 by Morsanyi et al. evaluated the prevalence rates of specific learning disorder in mathematics, gender differences, and comorbid conditions. The prevalence rate was 6%. They found persistent difficulties in reading (5.6%) and language difficulties in English (11.5%) and also found that they had other comorbid symptoms and disorders such as social, emotional, and behavioral difficulties, autism, or attention deficit hyperactivity disorder [8]. There is still no agreed definition of mathematics disability and are controversies between researchers based on cutoff decisions, specificity and gender differences. Prevalence rates are summarized in **Table 1**.

3. Comorbidity of specific learning disorder

In the prevalence studies of specific learning disorders, ADHD, which receives the most comorbidity and is the most studied disorder, should be considered [1, 48]. Two American national studies by the same researchers found 4% prevalence of comorbidity [17, 49]. DuPaul et al. reported this comorbidity rate as 18–60% and found that the incidence of SLD in ADHD patients was 7 times higher than that of the population [50]. Some clinical studies have reported extremely high prevalence rates of SLD as 70% or ADHD as 82.5% in comorbid cases [51, 52]. Genetic studies support that these two disorders may be associated with similar hereditary factors [53–55]. The high comorbidity between SLD and ADHD, inadequate SLD definitions, and different methods used in studies may have different results in evaluating the prevalence of SLD. And also symptoms of children diagnosed with SLD are more persistent when they have behavioral problems in the first years of school than with SLDs without ADHD or any comorbidity [56]. Therefore, early diagnosis and treatment interventions can significantly change the incidence and prevalence rates of SLD.

4. Gender differences of specific learning disorder

DSM-5 is stated that SLD is two to three times more prevalent in boys than in girls [1]. In 4 different epidemiologic studies including 9799 children from England, Wales, and New Zealand, boy/girl rates of reading difficulties were 21.6%/7.9%, 20.6%/9.8%, 17.6%/13.0%, and 18.0%/13.0%. In this study, reading and spelling deficits were not analyzed separately, so that it remained unresolved [12]. Landerl and Moll reported balanced gender ratios for reading (fluency) deficits but a disproportionate number of boys for spelling deficits in German population [34]. In a study of Moll et al., more problems in boys than girls for combined reading and spelling problems were identified, and when isolated spelling disorder was evaluated, gender ratios were found balanced [3]. According to these studies, dyslexia was found to be higher in boys than girls. The most common reported in the literature is that of no gender difference of mathematics disability [8, 29, 39, 42, 43, 45, 47]. The other studies reported higher prevalence of mathematics difficulties in girls [3, 32, 34, 45] or boys [31, 40, 46, 57]. And also some studies reported inconsistency findings. For example, Devine et al. reported that although there was no gender difference in the prevalence of math learning difficulties between boys and girls, mathematics difficulties were much more common for girls than for boys [47].

5. Conclusion

SLD is a multifactorial disorder which has in its etiology a genetic predisposition and family load, developmental and cognitive factors, language spoken, and environmental factors including the level of education and socioeconomic situation. Comorbidity with other mental disorders reveals more severe symptoms of it. And also if clinical and educational interventions are not performed, behavioral and emotional symptoms may accompany this diagnosis. The use of diagnostic criteria and structured scales, whether the disorder is a uniform or mixed type of disorder, the characteristics of the spoken language, and the assessment of environmental factors will help to determine the prevalence rate results and treatment interventions more specific. An educational approach and early intervention treatment after the awareness of SLD findings will reduce the difficulties that may arise with this disorder in the preschool period.

Conflict of interest

The authors declare no conflict of interest.

Author details

Işık Görker
Department of Child and Adolescent Psychiatry, Faculty of Medicine, Trakya University, Edirne, Turkey

*Address all correspondence to: isikgorker@gmail.com

References

[1] Association AP. Diagnostic and Statistical Manual of Mental Disorders Fifth Edition (DSM V). Washington DC: American Psychiatric Association; 2013

[2] Tannock R. Rethinking ADHD and LD in DSM-5: Proposed changes in diagnostic criteria. Journal of Learning Disabilities. 2013;**46**(1):5-25. DOI: 10.1177/0022219412464341

[3] Moll K, Kunze S, Neuhoff N, Bruder J, Schulte-Korne G. Specific learning disorder: Prevalence and gender differences. PLoS One. 2014;**9**(7):e103537. DOI: 10.1371/journal.pone.0103537

[4] Altarac M, Saroha E. Lifetime prevalence of learning disability among US children. Pediatrics. 2007;**119**(Supplement 1):S77-S83

[5] Choudhary M, Jain A, Chahar C, Singhal AK. A case control study on specific learning disorders in school going children in Bikaner city. Indian Journal of Pediatrics. 2012;**79**(11):1477-1481. DOI: 10.1007/s12098-012-0699-7

[6] Fluss J, Ziegler JC, Warszawski J, Ducot B, Richard G, Billard C. Poor reading in French elementary school: The interplay of cognitive, behavioral, and socioeconomic factors. Journal of Developmental and Behavioral Pediatrics. 2009;**30**(3):206-216. DOI: 10.1097/DBP.0b013e3181a7ed6c

[7] Gorker I, Bozatli L, Korkmazlar U, Yucel Karadag M, Ceylan C, Sogut C, et al. The probable prevalence and sociodemographic characteristics of specific learning disorder in primary school children in edirne. Noro Psikiyatri Arsivi. 2017;**54**(4):343-349. DOI: 10.5152/npa.2016.18054

[8] Morsanyi K, van Bers B, McCormack T, McGourty J. The prevalence of specific learning disorder in mathematics and comorbidity with other developmental disorders in primary school-age children. British Journal of Psychology. 2018;**109**(4):917-940. DOI: 10.1111/bjop.12322

[9] Rathore S, Mangal S, Agdi P, Rathore K, Nema R, Mahatma O. An overview on dyslexia and its treatment. Journal of Global Pharma Technology. 2010;**2**:18-25

[10] Sun Z, Zou L, Zhang J, Mo S, Shao S, Zhong R, et al. Prevalence and associated risk factors of dyslexic children in a middle-sized city of China: A cross-sectional study. PLoS One. 2013;**8**(2):e56688. DOI: 10.1371/journal.pone.0056688

[11] Vlachos F, Avramidis E, Dedousis G, Chalmpe M, Ntalla I, Giannakopoulou M. Prevalence and gender ratio of dyslexia in Greek adolescents and its association with parental history and brain injury. American Journal of Educational Research. 2013;**1**(1):22-25

[12] Rutter M, Caspi A, Fergusson D, Horwood LJ, Goodman R, Maughan B, et al. Sex differences in developmental reading disability: New findings from 4 epidemiological studies. Journal of the American Medical Association. 2004;**291**(16):2007-2012. DOI: 10.1001/jama.291.16.2007

[13] Alesi M, Rappo G, Pepi A. Self-esteem at school and self-handicapping in childhood: Comparison of groups with learning disabilities. Psychological Reports. 2012;**111**(3):952-962

[14] Association AP. Diagnostic and Statistical Manual of Mental Disorders 4th edn (DSM-IV). Washington, DC: APA; 2000

[15] Taanila A, Yliherva A, Kaakinen M, Moilanen I, Ebeling H. An epidemiological

study on Finnish school-aged children with learning difficulties and behavioural problems. International Journal of Circumpolar Health. 2011;**70**(1):59-71. DOI: 10.3402/ijch.v70i1.17799

[16] Whitsell LJ. Learning disorders as a school health problem—Neurological and psychiatric aspects. California Medicine. 1969;**111**(6):433

[17] Pastor PN, Reuben CA. Attention deficit disorder and learning disability: United States, 1997-98. Vital Health and Statistics. Data from the National Health Interview Survey: ERIC. 2002

[18] Silver LB. Developmental learning disorder. In: Lewis M, editor. Child and Adolescent Psychiatry Textbook. 3rd ed. Philadelphia: Lippincott Williams & Wilkins; 2002. pp. 621-629

[19] Yao B, Wu HR. Risk factors of learning disabilities in Chinese children in Wuhan. Biomedical and Environmental Sciences. 2003;**16**(4):392-397

[20] Al-Yagon M, Cavendish W, Cornoldi C, Fawcett AJ, Grunke M, Hung LY, et al. The proposed changes for DSM-5 for SLD and ADHD: International perspectives—Australia, Germany, Greece, India, Israel, Italy, Spain, Taiwan, United Kingdom, and United States. Journal of Learning Disabilities. 2013;**46**(1):58-72. DOI: 10.1177/0022219412464353

[21] Del'Homme M, Kim TS, Loo SK, Yang MH, Smalley SL. Familial association and frequency of learning disabilities in ADHD sibling pair families. Journal of Abnormal Child Psychology. 2007;**35**(1):55-62. DOI: 10.1007/s10802-006-9080-5

[22] Fortes IS, Paula CS, Oliveira MC, Bordin IA, de Jesus Mari J, Rohde LA. A cross-sectional study to assess the prevalence of DSM-5 specific learning disorders in representative school samples from the second to sixth grade in Brazil. European Child & Adolescent Psychiatry. 2016;**25**(2):195-207. DOI: 10.1007/s00787-015-0708-2

[23] Geary DC. Mathematical disabilities: Cognitive, neuropsychological, and genetic components. Psychological Bulletin. 1993;**114**(2):345-362. DOI: 10.1037/0033-2909.114.2.345

[24] Hecht SA, Torgesen JK, Wagner RK, Rashotte CA. The relations between phonological processing abilities and emerging individual differences in mathematical computation skills: A longitudinal study from second to fifth grades. Journal of Experimental Child Psychology. 2001;**79**(2):192-227

[25] Jordon NC, Kaplan D, Hanich LB. Achievement growth in children with learning difficulties in mathematics: Findings of a two-year longitudinal study. Journal of Educational Psychology. 2002;**94**(3):586

[26] Geary DC, Hoard MK. Numerical and arithmetical deficits in learning-disabled children: Relation to dyscalculia and dyslexia. Aphasiology. 2001;**15**(7):635-647

[27] Lagae L. Learning disabilities: Definitions, epidemiology, diagnosis, and intervention strategies. Pediatric Clinics of North America. 2008;**55**(6):1259-1268, vii. DOI: 10.1016/j.pcl.2008.08.001

[28] Badian NA. Dyscalculia and nonverbal disorders of learning. Progress in Learning Disabilities. 1983;**5**:235-264

[29] Lewis C, Hitch GJ, Walker P. The prevalence of specific arithmetic difficulties and specific reading difficulties in 9- to 10-year-old boys and

girls. Journal of Child Psychology and Psychiatry. 1994;**35**(2):283-292. DOI: 10.1111/j.1469-7610.1994.tb01162.x

[30] Miles T, Haslum M, Wheeler T. Gender ratio in dyslexia. Annals of Dyslexia. 1998;**48**(1):27-55

[31] Badian NA. Reading disability defined as a discrepancy between listening and reading comprehension: A longitudinal study of stability, gender differences, and prevalence. Journal of Learning Disabilities. 1999;**32**(2):138-148

[32] Dirks E, Spyer G, van Lieshout EC, de Sonneville L. Prevalence of combined reading and arithmetic disabilities. Journal of Learning Disabilities. 2008;**41**(5):460-473. DOI: 10.1177/0022219408321128

[33] von Aster M, Schweiter M, Weinhold Zulauf M. Rechenstörungen bei Kindern. Zeitschrift für Entwicklungspsychologie und Pädagogische Psychologie. 2007;**39**(2):85-96

[34] Landerl K, Moll K. Comorbidity of learning disorders: Prevalence and familial transmission. Journal of Child Psychology and Psychiatry. 2010;**51**(3):287-294. DOI: 10.1111/j.1469-7610.2009.02164.x

[35] Huc-Chabrolle M, Barthez MA, Tripi G, Barthelemy C, Bonnet-Brilhault F. Psychocognitive and psychiatric disorders associated with developmental dyslexia: A clinical and scientific issue. Encephale. 2010;**36**(2):172-179. DOI: 10.1016/j.encep.2009.02.005

[36] Dhanda A, Jagawat T. Prevalence and pattern of learning disabilities in school children. Delhi Psychiatry Journal. 2013;**16**(2):386-390

[37] Cappa C, Giulivi S, Schiliro A, Bastiani L, Muzio C, Meloni F. A screening on specific learning disorders in an Italian speaking high genetic homogeneity area. Research in Developmental Disabilities. 2015;**45-46**:329-342. DOI: 10.1016/j.ridd.2015.07.011

[38] Dalton P. Dyslexia & Dyscalculia. Parliamentary Office of Science and Technology. Postnote; 2004:226

[39] Mazzocco MM, Myers GF. Complexities in identifying and defining mathematics learning disability in the primary school-age years. Annals of Dyslexia. 2003;**53**(1):218-253. DOI: 10.1007/s11881-003-0011-7

[40] Barbaresi WJ, Katusic SK, Colligan RC, Weaver AL, Jacobsen SJ. Math learning disorder: Incidence in a population-based birth cohort, 1976-82, Rochester, Minn. Ambulatory Pediatrics. 2005;**5**(5):281-289. DOI: 10.1367/A04-209R.1

[41] Barahmand U. Arithmetic disabilities: Training in attention and memory enhances arithmetic ability. Research Journal of Biological Sciences. 2008;**3**(11):1305-1312

[42] Hein J, Bzufka MW, Neumärker K-J. The specific disorder of arithmetic skills. Prevalence studies in a rural and an urban population sample and their clinico-neuropsychological validation. European Child & Adolescent Psychiatry. 2000;**9**(2):S87-S101

[43] Desoete A, Roeyers H, De Clercq A. Children with mathematics learning disabilities in Belgium. Journal of Learning Disabilities. 2004;**37**(1):50-61. DOI: 10.1177/00222194040370010601

[44] Geary DC. Missouri longitudinal study of mathematical development and disability. BJEP Monograph Series II, Number 7-Understanding Number Development and Difficulties. 31:

British Psychological Society; 2010. pp. 31-49

[45] Gross-Tsur V, Manor O, Shalev RS. Developmental dyscalculia: Prevalence and demographic features. Developmental Medicine and Child Neurology. 1996;**38**(1):25-33. DOI: 10.1111/j.1469-8749.1996.tb15029.x

[46] Ramaa S, Gowramma I. A systematic procedure for identifying and classifying children with dyscalculia among primary school children in India. Dyslexia. 2002;**8**(2):67-85

[47] Devine A, Soltesz F, Nobes A, Goswami U, Szucs D. Gender differences in developmental dyscalculia depend on diagnostic criteria. Learning and Instruction. 2013;**27**:31-39. DOI: 10.1016/j.learninstruc.2013.02.004

[48] Pham AV, Riviere A. Specific learning disorders and ADHD: Current issues in diagnosis across clinical and educational settings. Current Psychiatry Reports. 2015;**17**(6):38. DOI: 10.1007/s11920-015-0584-y

[49] Pastor PN, Reuben CA. Diagnosed attention deficit hyperactivity disorder and learning disability: United States, 2004-2006. Data from the National Health Interview Survey. Vital and Health Statistics. Series 10, Number 237: ERIC; 2008

[50] DuPaul GJ, Volpe RJ. ADHD and learning disabilities: Research findings and clinical implications. Current Attention Disorders Reports. 2009;**1**(4):152

[51] Altay MA, Gorker I. Assessment of psychiatric comorbidity and WISC-R profiles in cases diagnosed with specific learning disorder according to DSM-5 criteria. Noro Psikiyatri Arsivi. 2018;**55**(2):127-134. DOI: 10.5152/npa.2017.18123

[52] Mayes SD, Calhoun SL, Crowell EW. Learning disabilities and ADHD: Overlapping spectrum disorders. Journal of Learning Disabilities. 2000;**33**(5):417-424

[53] Cheung CH, Frazier-Wood AC, Asherson P, Rijsdijk F, Kuntsi J. Shared cognitive impairments and aetiology in ADHD symptoms and reading difficulties. PLoS One. 2014;**9**(6):e98590. DOI: 10.1371/journal.pone.0098590

[54] Hong DS. Here/in this issue and there/abstract thinking: Learning disorders and ADHD: Are LDs getting the attention they deserve? Journal of the American Academy of Child and Adolescent Psychiatry. 2014;**53**(9):933

[55] Willcutt EG, Pennington BF, Smith SD, Cardon LR, Gayán J, Knopik VS, et al. Quantitative trait locus for reading disability on chromosome 6p is pleiotropic for attention-deficit/hyperactivity disorder. American Journal of Medical Genetics. 2002;**114**(3):260-268

[56] Sanson A, Prior M, Smart D. Reading disabilities with and without behaviour problems at 7-8 years: Prediction from longitudinal data from infancy to 6 years. Journal of child Psychology and Psychiatry. 1996;**37**(5):529-541

[57] Reigosa-Crespo V, Valdes-Sosa M, Butterworth B, Estevez N, Rodriguez M, Santos E, et al. Basic numerical capacities and prevalence of developmental dyscalculia: The Havana Survey. Developmental Psychology. 2012;**48**(1):123-135. DOI: 10.1037/a0025356

Chapter 3

Neural Correlates in Learning Disabilities

Misciagna Sandro

Abstract

In recent years, researchers have done significant advances on the study of learning disabilities in particular in terms of comprehension of cognitive and anatomical mechanisms. The understanding of neural mechanism of learning disabilities is useful for their management and cognitive treatment. The advent of functional neuroimaging methods has also identified anatomical networks and neurological learning systems that have contributed to knowledge of neurobiology of learning deficits. On the other side, neuropsychological assessment, with comprehensive test or specific cognitive tasks, has proved to be useful to analyze specific cognitive deficits to find potential targets of intervention for cognitive compensation. In this chapter the author summarizes major scientific advances in particular in the study of neuroanatomical mechanism based on structural and functional neuroimaging of children with learning disorders, developmental disorders, and language impairment, in particular with dyslexia which is one of the most common learning disabilities.

Keywords: learning disabilities, learning deficits, learning disorders, dyslexia, reading disorders, dyscalculia, math disorders, dysgraphia, text generation disorders, anatomical mechanism, neurobiology, neural mechanism, functional neuroimaging, anatomical networks, learning systems

1. Cognitive bases of learning disabilities

Learning disabilities have been studied by neuropsychological researchers over the past 50 years, so many scientific articles have been published on this topic.

The understanding of learning disorders has relevant implications both for assessment and cognitive interventions.

Early cases of children with learning disorders were described by an ophthalmologist who studied children with reading difficulties without brain lesions, so they considered these children as affected by "word blindness" [1].

Subsequently medical researchers used the term "dyslexia" to describe children with troubles in reading and spelling isolated words; they attributed dyslexia to a disorder of cerebral dominance for language [2]. Other authors used the term "learning disabilities" to refer to children with unexpected difficulties secondary to language disorders, differentiating learning disabilities from behavioral disorders and intellectual disabilities [3].

In the 1970s, neuropsychologists started a period of research to identify the cognitive bases of learning disabilities. They emphasized in particular the importance of profile interpretations for inferring brain dysfunction in learning disabilities [4].

Other researchers identified neuropsychological correlates of reading difficulties including finger agnosia [5], right–left confusion, auditory–visual integration [6], color-naming difficulties [7], or other language problems.

Some scientists hypothesized that learning disabilities could be related to a parietal lobe disorder [5] or to a developmental Gerstmann syndrome [8].

Some authors attributed reading difficulties to a maturational lag in brain development [9] or to language difficulties [10].

Other researchers criticized theories based on group comparison of single variables in favor of multivariate approaches [11]. This led to researches in which profile of neuropsychological tests were identified to better study the cognitive deficits of learning disabilities [12].

One of the most significance influences on the scientific understanding of learning disabilities was the "theory of speech processing" as a segmented signal of phonological representation [13]. According to this theory, phonological awareness is a metacognitive understanding of the sound structure of speech. The children learning to read must link the orthographic patterns of written language to the internal structure of speech to access the developing lexical system. This theory has been verified across languages that vary in the transparency of orthography and phonology [14].

These discoveries were important in the understanding of learning disabilities since a specific phonological awareness and cognitive skill was considered linked to decoding a specific academic skill, explaining success and failure in reading.

The differentiation of learning disabilities into academic domains produced an expansion of base researches about cognitive correlates and neurobiological factors related to cognitive domains of learning disabilities [15].

Thus learning disorders were separated into three principal domains and six subdomains:

1. Oral reading domains that occur at the level of word (*dyslexia*) and the level of text (*reading comprehension disorders*)

2. Math domains that could be computational (*dyscalculia*) or involve executive mathematical functions (*math problem-solving disorders*)

3. Written language domains that could involve basic skills needed for transcription (handwriting and spelling *dysgraphia*) and generating text in essays or stories *(text generation disorders*)

According to Pennington and Peterson, problems in these cognitive domains generate higher-order language, attentional, and executive disorders that affect oral and written language [16]. In other cases, these cognitive disorders are often comorbid with other behavioral traits, such as attention-deficit/hyperactivity disorders (ADHD) [17] or developmental language disorders [18].

Over the years, international researchers have mapped the framework of different sources of variability that influence learning disabilities [19] to help to establish the bases for effective interventions (**Figure 1**).

According to this framework, learning disabilities are related with neurobiological factors (brain structure and function, genetic factors) [15], cognitive processes (e.g., phonemic awareness), psychosocial factors (e.g., attention, anxiety, motivation), and environmental context (socioeconomic conditions, schooling, instruction, home environment).

Researchers have showed that intellectual quotient (IQ) is not predictive of learning disabilities [20], while processing speed deficits and working

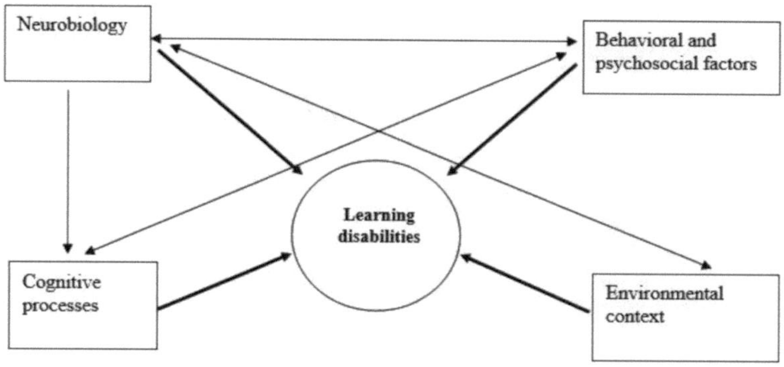

Figure 1.
Framework of different sources that influence learning disabilities.

memory are linked to learning disorders as well as comorbidity with ADHD [21]. Phonological awareness is also a strong predictor of failure or success in reading acquisition [22]. Time reading and spelling assessment could be used in the identification of dyslexia in more transparent languages [23], while vocabulary tasks, listening comprehension, and attention/executive function tasks could be used to study text-level disorders [24]. The learning abilities of individual with dyslexia have been examined using serial reaction time measures, revealing a moderate effect that indicates that automatization of learning is impaired in this disorder [25].

Neuropsychological studies have also suggested neurological and functional distinction between different types of learning: procedural learning system is involved in implicit learning and impaired in individual with specific language impairments [26], while declarative learning system were argued to be relatively intact. Children with dyslexia appear to have difficulty extracting structure from novel sequences in artificial grammar learning paradigms [27] and difficulties in making judgments about grammaticality, confirming that implicit learning processes are involved in dyslexic patients. Prominent difficulties in procedural learning in sequence-based tasks and relative preservation on declarative and nonsequential procedural learning may explain why individuals with learning disabilities have more difficulties in language tasks in which they have to extract and produce sequential information.

Math disabilities without reading difficulties are very common as comorbidity in children with learning disabilities [28]. Attention, working memory, and phonological processing are also overlapped with math problem-solving disorders, even if less studied than computational skills [29]. These findings support the view that mathematical abilities involve multiple cognitive processes and that math disorders reflect more generalized cognitive difficulties [30]. Executive functions that affect self-regulation are relevant for text generation disorders [31].

2. Neurobiological bases of learning disabilities

In recent years, research on brain structure and cerebral function of children with learning disabilities has taken advantage of new noninvasive structural and functional technologies.

Most studies have been focused on the study of dyslexia using neuroimaging studies (magnetic resonance imaging (MRI)) or functional studies (electroencephalography, event-related potentials, functional magnetic resonance imaging, positron emission tomography) [32].

Studies based on functional neuroimaging have identified a network of three regions localized in the left hemisphere mediating word reading:

1. A sublexical dorsal stream localized in temporoparietal areas

2. A lexical ventral stream localized in occipitotemporal region

3. A cerebral area in the left inferior frontal lobe underactivated or overactivated by temporoparietal or occipitotemporal regions (**Figure 2**)

This network, universal across different languages and orthographies [33], consists of a dorsal and ventral component that operates in parallel, connecting to the inferior frontal gyrus. The dorsal stream is associated with sublexical route to word meaning, consistent with word reading, while the ventral stream is specialized for visual processing of orthographic patterns [34]. The fusiform gyrus is considered an area that mediates word recognition with direct access to semantic regions in inferior temporal regions [35].

Researches based on functional MRI have demonstrated that the development of ventral system is dependent on exposure to print and that in children this system shows reorganization with explicit instructions in reading [36].

Quantitative analyses of MRI have shown reduced volume of the network of pre-scholars before the onset of formal reading instructions [37].

The dorsal and ventral pathways have resulted similar pattern of activation in children with word-level learning disabilities when compared with children developing reading comprehension learning disabilities (RCLD). In contrast the group of children with RCLD showed reduced deactivation of the left angular, left inferior frontal, and left hippocampal and parahippocampal gyri [38]. In other structural studies conducted on adolescent with RCLD, researchers found reduced gray matter in the right frontal regions, explaining their executive function disorders [39].

Functional MRI studies in adults have found that language learning also implicates corticostriatal and hippocampal systems. These structures are connected to each other as well as to the cortex and to other subcortical structures (**Figure 3**).

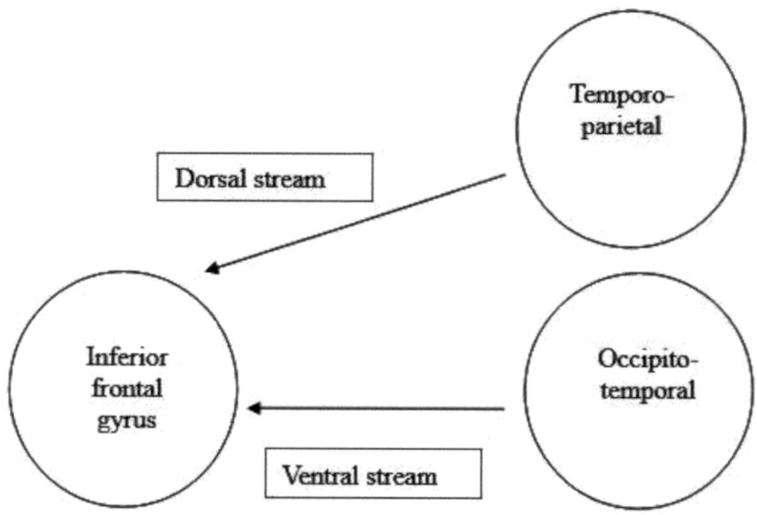

Figure 2.
Cerebral network that influences word reading.

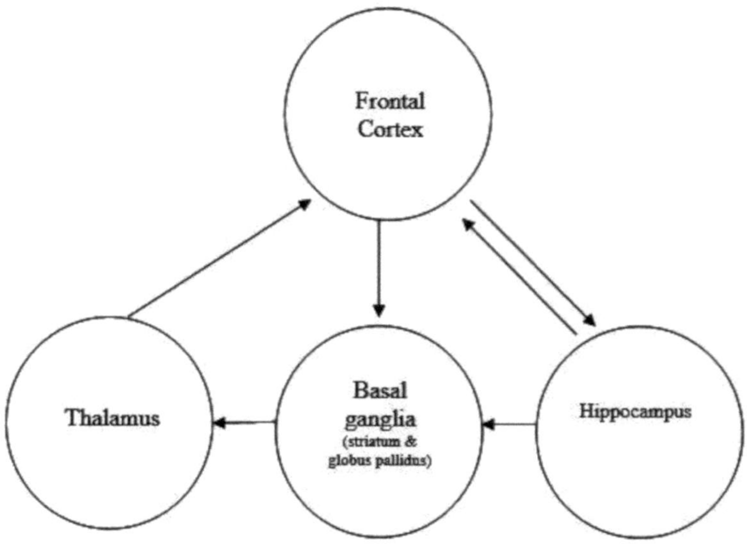

Figure 3.
Corticostriatal and hippocampal learning networks that influence language learning.

Functional interactions between these regions have been described during learning processes [40]. Consequently, changes in functional neural activity in one of these regions during language learning might reflect a local change of a complex learning network. The frontal cortex and basal ganglia appear to be relevant in learning the phonology and grammar of a language [41]. The hippocampus is also necessary in word learning; in fact, in fMRI studies, the hippocampus results to be activated during the process of learning new vocabularies [42] and during encoding processes related to words [43].

The ventral striatum (nucleus accumbens) is activated in learning novel words [44], while the dorsal striatum responds to feedback in verbal paired-associated tasks [45]. Abnormalities in the striatum have been seen also in children with language disorders [46]. Some studies suggest a reduction of volume of the caudate nucleus in children with specific language and learning impairment [47], while others have reported increases in caudate nucleus volume [48]. Functional studies conducted on adults with dyslexia show hyperactivation of the striatum, not seen in children with dyslexia, suggesting to be a compensatory mechanism in adulthood. Structural network analysis in children with a higher risk for dyslexia and other reading difficulties have showed that the hippocampus, temporal lobe, and putamen are less strongly connected in these individuals [49].

Studies conducted on children with math disabilities have found disorders of connectivity in temporoparietal and inferior parietal white matter [50].

Researchers have not found consistent structural differences across all studies in dyslexic patients, probably since this disorder is the result of a combination of multiple risk factors including motor, oral language, phonological disorders, and executive deficits [51].

Functional neuroimaging studies on numerical processing and mental arithmetic have also demonstrated the existence of a neural network [52], connecting frontotemporal regions with three left parietal circuits: superior parietal, intraparietal, and inferior parietal (**Figure 4**). This network is characterized by increased activity in children with math learning disabilities [53].

Other reports have demonstrated that specific cerebellar regions contribute to cognitive functions in children with learning disorders in particular with verbal short-term memory deficits [54], reading development [55], or in general to cognitive, emotional, and behavioral functions [56].

According to the cerebellar deficit hypothesis, specific regions of the cerebellum are functionally connected with cerebral reading network [57].

The reading-related cerebral regions that result to have functional connectivity with the cerebellum are supposed to be three: the inferior frontal junction (IFJ), the inferior parietal lobule (IPL), and the middle temporal gyrus (MTG) (**Figure 5**).

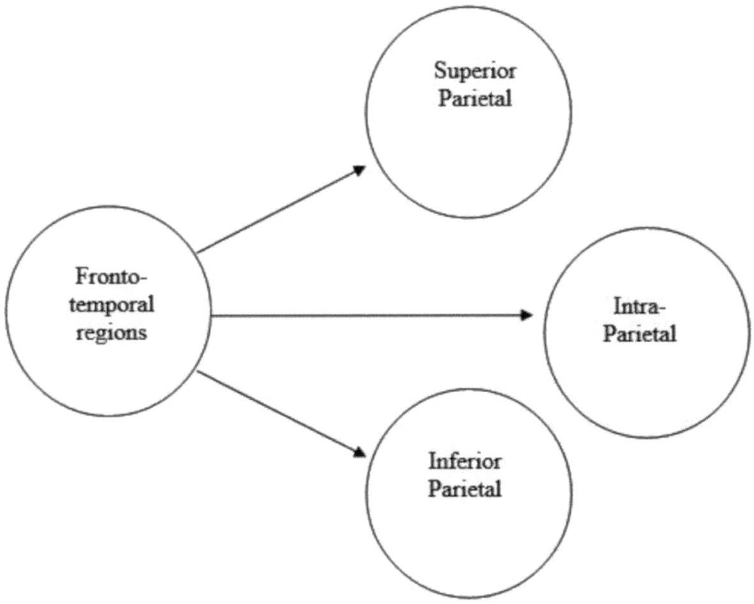

Figure 4.
Cerebral network that influences numerical processing.

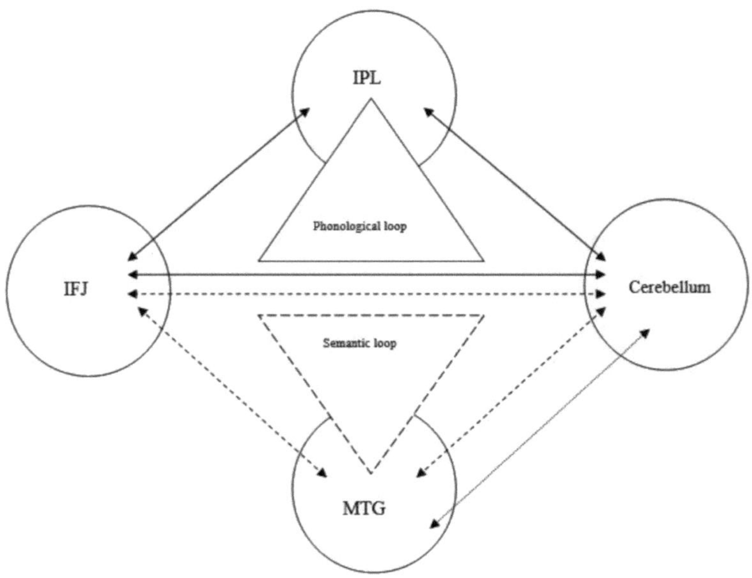

Figure 5.
Cerebro-cerebellar network that influences reading processing.

An analysis on connectivity has demonstrated three distinct sets of connections between cerebral and cerebellar regions. The first set of connections consist of a connection between IFJ and IPL that converges to a region in the right lateral posterior inferior cerebellum and is supposed to have a phonological role. The second set of connections consist of a connection between IFJ and MTG, which converges to a region in the right posterior superior cerebellum and is supposed to have a semantic role. The third set consist of a functional connectivity between MTG region and lateral anterior region of the cerebellum. There is not a common functional terminology for the third set of connections [55].

3. Conclusions

Studies conducted on children with learning disabilities, in particular with dyslexia, have shown an involvement in the function of cerebral areas and systems relevant in cognitive process about speech and learning (summarized in **Table 1**).

As evidenced in **Table 1**, structural or functional abnormalities of cerebral systems, localized in particular in the left hemisphere, in corticostriatal systems, and in cerebro-cerebellar connections, support the hypothesis of the existence of cerebral networks that can explain learning disorders.

These cerebral areas have an important impact on the development of learning and different aspects of language such as phonological and morpho-syntactic aspects.

Cognitive function	Cerebral areas	Hemisphere
Word reading	Dorsal stream: temporoparietal	Left
Visual processing of orthographic patterns	Ventral stream: occipitotemporal	Left
Lexical functions	Occipitotemporal	Left
Orthographic function	Inferior frontal gyrus	Left
Word recognition	Fusiform gyrus	Left
Semantic functions	Inferior temporal regions	Left
Reading comprehension	Both dorsal and ventral streams	Left
Executive functions	Frontal regions	Left and right
General language learning	Corticostriatal and hippocampal systems	Left
Learning of phonology and grammar	Frontal cortex and basal ganglia	Left
Word learning	Hippocampus	Left
Learning of new words	Ventral striatum (nucleus accumbens)	Left
Feedback in verbal paired-associated tasks	Dorsal striatum	Left
Numerical processing and mental arithmetic	Fronto-temporoparietal regions	Left
Math learning	Fronto-temporoparietal regions	Left
Verbal short-term memory	Cerebellum	Right?
Reading development	Cerebellum	Right?

Table 1.
Cerebral areas that influence cognitive learning processes.

However, there is a need to develop further longitudinal studies, conducted on children with learning disabilities, to explore cerebral anatomical and functional alterations during development and their correlation with specific pattern of learning disabilities.

Further progress in understanding the nature and specific components of learning difficulties in children will allow us to develop future specific targets and rehabilitative strategies of intervention.

Author details

Misciagna Sandro
Belcolle Hospital, Viterbo, Italy

*Address all correspondence to: sandromisciagna@yahoo.it

References

[1] Hinshelwood J. Word-blindness and visual memory. Lancet. 1895:1564-1570

[2] Orton S. Specific reading disability—Strephosymbolia. Journal of the American Medical Association. 1928;**90**:1095-1099

[3] Kirk SA. Behavioral diagnosis and remediation of learning disabilities. In: Conference on Exploring Problems of the Perceptually Handicapped Child, Vol. 1. 1963. pp. 1-23

[4] Rourke BP. Brain–behavior relationships in children with learning disabilities: A research program. American Psychologist. 1975;**30**:911-920

[5] Benton AL. Development dyslexia: Neurological aspects. In: Friedlander WJ, editor. Advances in Neurology. Vol. 7. New York: Raven Press; 1975. pp. 1-47

[6] Belmont L, Birch HG, Belmont I. Auditory-visual intersensory processing and verbal mediation. The Journal of Nervous and Mental Disease. 1968;**147**(6):562-569

[7] Geschwind N, Fusillo M. Color-naming defects in association with Alexia. Archives of Neurology. 1966;**15**:137-146

[8] Kinsbourne M, Warrington EK. Developmental factors in reading and writing backwardness. British Journal of Psychology. 1963;**54**:145-156

[9] Satz P, Sparrow S. Specific developmental dyslexia: A theoretical formulation. In: Bakker DF, Satz P, editors. Specific Reading Disability: Advances in Theory and Method. Rotterdam: Rotterdam University Press; 1970. pp. 17-39

[10] Vellutino FR. Toward an understanding of dyslexia: Psychological factors in specific reading disability. In: Benton AL, Pearl D, editors. Dyslexia. New York: Oxford University Press; 1978. pp. 61-112

[11] Doehring DG. The tangled web of behavioral research on developmental dyslexia. In: Benton AL, Pearl D, editors. Dyslexia. New York: Oxford University Press; 1978. pp. 123-137

[12] Rourke BP, editor. Neuropsychology of Learning Disabilities: Essentials of Subtype Analysis. New York: Guilford Press; 1985

[13] Liberman IY. Basic research in speech and lateralization of language. Bulletin of the Orton Society. 1971;**21**:72-87

[14] Ziegler JC, Goswami U. Reading acquisition, developmental dyslexia, and skilled reading across languages: A psycho-linguistic grain size theory. Psychological Bulletin. 2005;**131**:3-29

[15] Fletcher JM, Grinorenko EL. Neuropsychology of learning disabilities: The past and the future. Journal of the International Neuropsychological Society. 2017;**23**(9-10):930-940

[16] Pennington BF, Peterson R. Neurodevelopmental disorders: Learning disorders. In: Tasman A, Kay J, Lieberman JA, First MB, Riba MR, editors. Psychiatry. 4th ed. Chichester, UK: John Wiley & Sons; 2015

[17] Mahone M, Denckla MB. Attention-deficit/hyperactivity disorder. Journal of the International Neuropsychological Association. 2017;**23**(9-10):916-929

[18] Pennington BF. Diagnosing Learning Disorders: A Neuropsychological Framework. 2nd ed. New York: Guilford; 2009

[19] Fletcher JM, Lyon GR, Fuchs LS, Barnes MA. Learning Disabilities: From Identification to Intervention. 2nd ed. New York: Guilford Press; 2007. p. 324

[20] Stuebing KK, Fletcher JM, LeDoux JM, Lyon GR, Shaywitz SE, Shaywitz BA. Validity of IQ-discrepancy classifications of reading disabilities: A meta-analysis. American Educational Research Journal. 2002;**39**:469-518

[21] McGrath LM, Pennington BF, Shanahan MA, Santerre-Lemmon LE, Barnard HD, Willcutt EG, et al. A multiple deficit model of reading disability and attention-deficit/hyperactivity disorder: Searching for shared cognitive deficits. Journal of Child Psychology and Psychiatry. 2011;**52**(5):547-557

[22] Melby-Lervåg M, Lyster SAH, Hulme C. Phonological skills and their role in learning to read: A meta-analytic review. Psychological Bulletin. 2012;**138**:322-352

[23] Wimmer H, Mayringer H. Dysfluent reading in the absence of spelling difficulties: A specific disability in regular orthographies. Journal of Educational Psychology. 2002;**94**:272-277

[24] Cain K, Barnes MA. Reading comprehension. In: Parrila RK, Cain K, Compton DL, editors. Theories of Reading Development. Amsterdam: John Benjamins; 2017. pp. 257-282

[25] Nicolson RI, Fawcett AJ. Procedural learning difficulties: Reuniting the developmental disorders? Trends in Neurosciences. 2007;**30**:135-141

[26] Ullman MT, Pierpont EI. Specific language impairment is not specific to language: The procedural deficit hypothesis. Cortex. 2005;**41**:399-433

[27] Pavlidou EV et al. Do children with developmental dyslexia have impairments in implicit learning? Dyslexia. 2010;**16**:143-161

[28] Willcutt EG, Petrill SA, Wu S, Boada R, DeFries JC, Olson RK, et al. Comorbidity between reading disability and math disability: Concurrent psychopathology, functional impairment, and neuropsychological functioning. Journal of Learning Disabilities. 2013;**46**:500-516

[29] Fuchs LS, Fuchs D, Hamlett CL, Lambert W, Stuebing K, Fletcher JM. Problem-solving and computational skill: Are they shared or distinct aspects of mathematical cognition? Journal of Educational Psychology. 2008;**100**:30-47

[30] Geary DC. Early foundations for mathematics learning and their relations to learning disabilities. Current Directions in Psychological Science. 2013;**22**(1):23-27

[31] Berninger VW. Understanding the graphia in developmental dysgraphia: A developmental neuropsychological perspective for disorders in producing written language. In: Dewey D, Tupper D, editors. Developmental Motor Disorders: A Neuropsychological Perspective. New York: Guilford Press; 2004. pp. 189-233

[32] Rumsey JM, Zametkin AJ, Andreason P, Hanchan AP, Hamburger SD, Aquino T, et al. Normal activation of frontotemporal language cortex in dyslexia, as measured with oxygen 15 positron emission tomography. Archives of Neurology. 1994;**51**:27-38

[33] Paulesu E, Démonet JF, Fazio F, McCrory E, Chanoine V, Brunswick N, et al. Dyslexia: Cultural diversity and biological unity. Science. 2001;**291**:2165-2167

[34] Vogel AC, Petersen SE, Schlaggar BL. The VWFA: It's not just

for words anymore. Frontiers in Human Neuro-science. 2014;**8**:1-10

[35] Dehaene S. Reading in the Brain: The New Science of how we Read. London: Penguin; 2009

[36] Dehaene S, Cohen L, Morais J, Kolinsky R. Illiterate to literate: Behavioural and cerebral changes induced by reading acquisition. Nature Reviews Neuroscience. 2015;**16**:234-244

[37] Raschle NM, Becker BLC, Smith S, Fehlbaum LV, Wang Y, Gaab N. Investigating the influences of language delay and/or familial risk for dyslexia on brain structure in 5-year-olds. Cerebral Cortex. 2017;**27**:764-776

[38] Cutting LE, Clements-Stephens A, Pugh KR, Burns S, Cao A, Pekar JJ, et al. Not all reading disabilities are dyslexia: Distinct neurobiology of specific comprehension deficits. Brain Connectivity. 2013;**3**(2):199-211

[39] Bailey S, Hoeft F, Aboud K, Cutting L. Anomalous gray matter patterns in specific reading comprehension deficit are independent of dyslexia. Annals of Dyslexia. 2016;**66**:256-274

[40] Packard MG, Knowlton BJ. Learning and memory functions of the basal ganglia. Annual Review of Neuroscience. 2002;**25**:563-593

[41] Karuza EA et al. The neural correlates of statistical learning in a word segmentation task: An fMRI study. Brain and Language. 2013;**127**:46-54

[42] Breitenstein C et al. Hippocampus activity differentiates good from poor learners of a novel lexicon. NeuroImage. 2005;**25**:958-968

[43] Wing EA et al. Neural correlates of retrieval-based memory enhancement: An fMRI study of the testing effect. Neuropsychologia. 2013;**51**:2360-2370

[44] Ripollés P et al. The role of reward in word learning and its implications for language acquisition. Current Biology. 2014;**24**:2606-2611

[45] Tricomi E, Fiez JA. Information content and reward processing in the human striatum during performance of a declarative memory task. Cognitive, Affective, & Behavioral Neuroscience. 2011;**12**:361-372

[46] Krishnan S, Watkins KE, Bishop DVM. Neurobiological basis of language learning difficulties. Trends in Cognitive Sciences. 2016;**20**(9):701-714. DOI: 10.1016/j.tics.2016.06.012

[47] Jernigan TL et al. Cerebral structure on magnetic resonance imaging in language and learning-impaired children. Archives of Neurology. 1991;**48**:539-545

[48] Soriano-Mas C et al. Age-related brain structural alterations in children with specific language impairment. Human Brain Mapping. 2009;**30**:1626-1636

[49] Hosseini SMH et al. Topological properties of large-scale structural brain networks in children with familial risk for reading difficulties. NeuroImage. 2013;**71**:260-274

[50] Matejko AA, Ansari D. Drawing connections between white matter and numerical and mathematical cognition: A literature review. Neuroscience & Biobehavioral Reviews. 2015;**48**:35-52

[51] Thompson PA et al. Developmental dyslexia: Predicting individual risk. Journal of Child Psychology and Psychiatry. 2015;**56**:976-987

[52] Venkatraman V, Ansari D, Chee MW. Neural correlates of symbolic and non-symbolic arithmetic. Neuropsychologia. 2005;**43**(5):744-753

[53] Iuculano T, Rosenberg-Lee M, Richardson J, Tenison C, Fuchs L,

Supekar K, et al. Cognitive tutoring induces widespread neuroplasticity and remediates brain function in children with mathematical learning disabilities. Nature Communications. 2015;**6**:8453

[54] Misciagna S, Iuvone L, Mariotti P, Silveri MC. Verbal short-term memory and cerebellum: Evidence from a patient with congenital cerebellar vermis hypoplasia. Neurocase. 2009:1-6

[55] Alvarez TA, Fiez JA. Current perspectives on the cerebellum and reading development. Neuroscience and Biobehavioral Reviews. 2018;**92**:55-66

[56] Misciagna S. Cerebellar contribution to cognitive, emotional and behavioral functions in children with cerebellar abnormalities. Developmental Medicine and Child Neurology. 2011;**53**(12):1075-1076

[57] Nicolson RI, Fawcett AJ, Dean P. Developmental dyslexia: The cerebellar deficit hypothesis. Trends in Neurosciences. 2001;**24**:508-511

Section 2

Differential Diagnosis of Common Learning Disabilities

Chapter 4

Identifying and Remediating Dyslexia in Kindergarten and the Foundation Year

Diane Montgomery

Abstract

Dyslexia is a learning disability found across the ability range. It is an unexpected failure to learn to read and spell despite conventional classroom instruction. It is usually identified at about 7 years of age or beyond when the dyslexic fails to learn to read. The incidence varies in different countries in different languages and with teaching methods. This research presents a new method for the identification of dyslexia by the Reception or Kindergarten teacher as part of everyday teaching. The method uses a child's freeform writing and a checklist that identifies a critical borderline point that must be reached if the child is to become literate. In order to overcome any difficulty, a specific intervention was identified and a training technique was introduced in a Reception Year cohort (N = 175 children). It was based upon previous research that found dyslexia was caused by a unique deficit that prevented them from developing early phonological awareness in the normal course of learning. The intervention strategy also enabled disadvantaged learners to catch up with more advantaged peers and close the 11-month learning gap found in the national statistics. Their Key stage 1 school SATs showed 30% uplift 3 years later.

Keywords: dyslexia, disadvantage, kindergarten, reception year, intervention, remediation

1. Introduction

Dyslexia is an unexpected difficulty in learning to read and spell in relation to age and ability by the methods normally used in classrooms. In the modern era it has become a serious problem for large numbers of people as education has extended and demanded they become literate. Dyslexia is sometimes accompanied by and made worse by handwriting difficulties (dysgraphia), and whilst most dyslexics do eventually learn to read when given specialist tuition as adults, they still have residual spelling problems.

Because English is an opaque not a transparent language system, there are larger numbers of dyslexics in countries where English is the home language. Transparent languages such as Italian, Turkish and Spanish have a one-to-one correspondence between the sounds of the language (phonemes) and its written symbols (graphemes), and they are said to be 'regular' in this respect. English on the other hand has only a 40% phonemic regularity, and the rest is derived from its history with other languages mainly Norse, Anglo-Saxon, Greek, Latin and Norman French.

To accommodate this knowledge, 15 basic words and the rules that govern them can reveal how to spell 20,000 English words correctly [1]. But it is first of all an understanding of the alphabetic principle and how it is used that is crucial. It is this, with which Reception and Kindergarten learners have to cope.

Arabic, a Semitic language, with 33 phonemes is also a transparent language [2] and has been widely adapted to various other languages such as Urdu, Farsi and Kurdish. It was the Phoenicians in their Semitic language who were thought to have invented the alphabetic system to facilitate and record their trading negotiations [3]. This alphabetic principle is thought to have been invented just once about 2700 years ago and could probably only have occurred in the Semitic language because it was consonantal and did not have vowels; they were imported later by the Greeks. As will be explained it is unlikely that a dyslexic could have invented it.

The incidence of dyslexia in the UK, according to the British Dyslexia Association [4], is 10% of which 4% are severe cases. In some disadvantaged groups, the incidence can be as large as 19% [5]. It was also found that there were hidden populations of dyslexics who had learned to read but still had severe spelling problems especially with new and technical vocabulary. These amounted to one-third of cohorts in the disadvantaged areas. The result is that the poor spellers and writers underachieve at school and then at university. Their talents may lie hidden for many years. There is also a group that has learned to read often self-taught but have dyslexic spelling problems, and this has been termed 'dysorthographia'. Research and practice with this range of dyslexics over four decades formed the basis for the present studies.

2. Background theory and research

The research of Chall [6, 7] demonstrated that if teachers initially employed a purely visual system of reading teaching (paired associate memorising) called 'Look and Say', 4% of the learners became dyslexic. If however they were taught from the outset by a purely phonic system, the dyslexia rate was about 1–1.5% ([8]; SED (Scottish Education Department) The Education of Pupils with Learning Difficulties in Primary and Secondary Schools. A progress Report by HMI Edinburgh: HMSO 1978; [9, 10]). Over time UK Governments' encouragement to use 'mixed methods' and then 'Phonics First' [11] have met with limited success.

Over the same period research into the psychological processes involved in becoming literate, and literacy teaching have followed a similar path. The emphasis is placed on learning to read, and reading development has dominated both practice and research, whilst spelling was marginalised until recently. There have however been threads that can be traced showing that spelling is more important to learning to read than has previously been considered by many researchers and would repay more detailed investigation.

For example, although dyslexia research on a vast scale has centred upon the reading difficulties, both Chomsky [12] and Clay [13] found that children's first impulse was to write not read. When asked to write a message or story, the children picked up a pen and made 'marks on paper' and 'read' it back. When asked to read a storybook, they said they could not do so because they had not yet been taught to. It was when marks on paper such as these began to be studied that a range of levels of marks were observed. These went from scribbles and lines to letters and words carrying a decipherable message although not quite with traditional spelling. Occasionally there were cases of 5-year-olds entering school or Kindergarten who had learned to read and write self-taught, and they were not necessarily those with the highest of IQs [14].

'My little sister is in bed because she is having her tonsils out'.

Examples such as the writing of Faye above were collected after she had spent 1 month in the Reception class. The teachers said the children could not read or write free-form; although some could copy write, none could read as they had only just begun to teach them. The teachers were astonished at what some of the children already knew about writing. The error patterns may give a significant profile of a child's knowledge about the alphabetic system that has been picked up incidentally in a word-filled world and classroom. Disadvantaged learners would be disadvantaged in this respect as their parents might not share books and reading with them or give them pens and pencils to hold and make drawings. Once in school they could be expected to catch up, but what about dyslexics?

Figure 2 shows a dyslexic's lack of sound-symbol knowledge after a year and a half in school. He uses letters from his name (before condition), but his message is not readable. He shows some knowledge of word structure and leaves spaces between his 'words'. He has not been systematically taught phonics. However after 6 x 20 minute lessons on the dyslexia programme Teaching Reading Through Spelling (TRTS) [15], his new message is readable.

'I went to my nannys and I went hma anB hta my pna anB I sat up Lt anB Wto tave'.

'I went to my nanny's and I went home and had my dinner and I sat up late and watched TV'.

He has 'cracked the alphabetic code' although as yet he does not know all the sounds and their symbols. Some whole words from daily copy writing are now 'patched in'. The school did not permit joined up writing until the children were in Year 3! The rest of the pupils in Steven's class had learned to read and write to varying degrees, and even he had had extra individual reading coaching sessions, but after all this he had made no progress. Fortunately for him his teacher wanted to try the TRTS system, and after six sessions he had made significant progress at last—he had 'cracked the alphabetic code'.

The success of the TRTS sessions was because it used a multisensory-articulatory-phonological-training (MAPT) system, whereas traditional phonics systems use just multisensory phonics training, that is they combine writing the grapheme with saying its sound. MAPT focuses the attention on the 'feel' of the phoneme in the mouth as it is said and written. This means that the phoneme and grapheme that are regarded as abstract perceptual units [16] are linked by a concrete articulatory cue. These are most clear for the consonants, the vowels are more open mouthed with different placing, and it is noticeable that in the literacy acquisition phase, beginners identify and mainly write the consonants. As they progress they map more correct spelling versions onto this structure [17], and this can be seen in both the **Figures 1** and **2** examples above. As beginners try to spell, they can often be seen mouthing the words as they do so presumably to recall the links. As early as 1932, Monroe [18] had pointed out the importance for early readers and writers of articulating, subvocalising and mouthing the sounds of the letters.

The reason for introducing an articulation awareness (AA) training element was derived from earlier research in which it was found that in cohorts of dyslexics going through a specialist remedial teaching centre, an AA deficit was evident. When this was put to an experimental test, the following results were obtained:

Table 1 shows that spelling age matched controls and dyslexics performed well on phoneme segmentation tasks but differed significantly (p 0.01) on articulation awareness test items. Dyslexics on the waiting list to enter the remedial centre who were age matched as near as possible performed significantly poorly on both PS and AA tests [1, 19, 20].

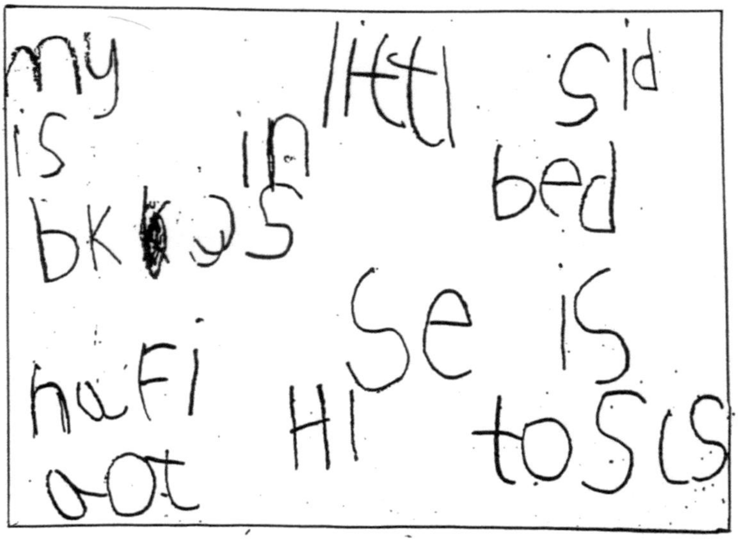

Figure 1.
Faye: 5 years 1 month.

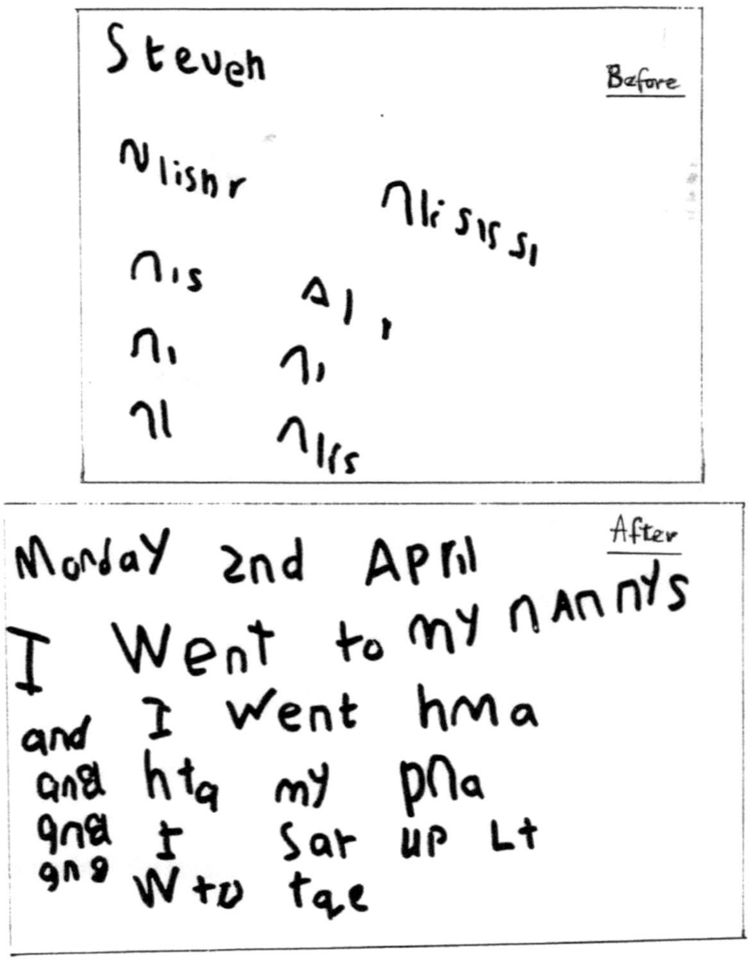

Figure 2.
Steven' writing aged 6.5 years in the 'Look and Say' era.

Dyslexia is currently regarded in the majority of cases as a verbal processing difficulty with particular problems in the area of phonological processing [21–24]. It is the problem that at least 90 per cent of dyslexics appear to present. On the basis of the research in **Table 1**, it was hypothesised that the phonological processing deficits might be caused by an underlying articulation awareness problem that prevented or delayed the learning of symbol-sound associations especially during implicit learning processes. It would mean that attention to a four-way system of VAKs principles should be followed rather than the three-way multisensory system used by most remedial teachers that omitted the kinaesthetic aspects of speech (**Figure 3**).

Reading and spelling development in dyslexics was analysed by Frith [25] as a process moving through three stages from logographic, to alphabetic and to orthographic based on the errors they made. She divided each stage into two further steps in which sometimes reading and sometimes spelling were the pacemakers. She explained that dyslexic children typically have difficulties moving from an early phase of acquisition in which reading is visually based (logographic) on the alphabetic phase when children are able to use letter-sound associations for both reading and spelling. This can be seen in the writing of Steven in **Figure 2**. In the 'before' condition, he can be seen to be stuck in the orthographic phase. With the specific MAPT training technique used in the early part of the TRTS programme, he makes the articulatory connections and can begin to use them to generate new words and enters the alphabetic phase. His developing skills in this respect can be seen in the second piece of writing after he writes some well-practised words.

At a later stage, some dyslexics fail to move from the alphabetic phase to the orthographic phase where reading and spelling were thought by Frith to be automatic and considered to be independent of sound. This condition is seen in many

	Nos	Reading Age	Spelling Age	PS (15)	Artic Aw (10)	IQ	Chron Age
Controls	84	8.61	8.02	11.94	7.75	110.03	7.94
Dyslexics on TRTS	114	7.95	7.62	10.27	4.31	110.43	12.90
Dyslexics waiting	30	6.71	6.0	4.13	5.87	112.67	8.97

Key: PS, phoneme segmentation (sing minus 's' gives 'ing', etc.). A 15-item test.
AA, articulation awareness. Test of 10 items.

Table 1.
Mean scores on phoneme segmentation (PS) and articulation awareness (AA).

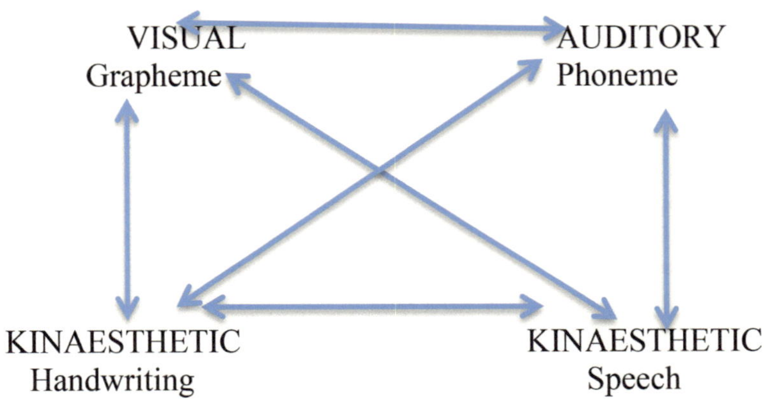

Figure 3.
To show the four-way multisensory VAK links.

adult dyslexics. Traditionally dyslexia has been identified in the alphabetic phase after a long delayed start when they are at least 2 years below the literacy level of peers. This level is not consistent with their age and ability. Various forms of intervention 'in class' then 'one-to-one additional support' may have been given and still have failed to bring them at least up to grade level. They are three-time failures by this time and often confused and upset. Even then an official diagnosis and funding support for specialist tuition might only be obtained just before entry to secondary school. Even so the remedial provision may not be adequate so although the dyslexic may begin to develop phonological awareness and start reading, he or she may never catch up with peers. To catch up means that they must make a 2-year literacy progress in each year of the specialist programme [23]. A meta-analysis of programme outcomes showing which are successful may be found in Montgomery [5, 26].

When dyslexia is identified in the early school years, remedial teachers report that it is easier to remediate. An extensive survey of 10,000 cases by Goldberg and Shiffman [27] had established this although they found that residual spelling errors remained.

Thus far a system to identify and remediate dyslexia in the early years by targeting sound-symbol correspondence development in the Logographic phase had not been developed. The Logographic phase is the literacy acquisition stage, the task of the Reception (Foundation Year) or Kindergarten learner. Sound-symbol correspondence is important for decoding unknown words during reading and for encoding for spelling, and this is why there was an emphasis in the United Kingdom on 'Phonics first' [11] and in the Early Years Foundation Stage guidelines [28] in the presence of a 'Look and Say' ethos.

This research however was pointing to a new direction for dyslexia investigation and remediation, and this was the role and meaning of children's early marks on paper in the logographic phase.

3. The research on early marks on paper

Normal spellers according to Gentry [29] also go through a logographic phase, but he found that there are two steps in it. The first step was pre-communicative in which marks and scribble were made as children 'wrote' their stories. This was followed by a prephonetic step in which there were invented or creative spellings in which a single letter or 'phone' or several letters might represent a word. Surprisingly research with dyslexics by Liberman [30], Bryant and Bradley [31] and Bourassa and Treiman [32] found the same characteristics, but there was a failure to move into the prephonetic stage. This was detectible not in their reading but in their attempts to write [1, 10]. Once the literacy journey had begun although several years later the reading and spelling errors of the dyslexics did not differ significantly from those of normal writers [19, 32].

In literacy learning, we have a situation in which normal readers and spellers learn sound-symbol correspondence implicitly or when specifically taught in Reception and some even arrive with that knowledge, and dyslexics who do not. Surely their problem must be detectable at an early stage as they fail to move into the prephonetic stage? This was the basic research question.

Previous research had found such a system was necessary for dyslexics because they appeared to have an articulation awareness deficit [1, 19]. This was potentially an observable sign of the neurological problem found in the 'pick up' systems by James and Engelhardt [33]. Their research showed during fMRI scanning that when preliterate 5-year-olds traced, printed or typed letters and shapes and then were shown images of these stimuli, a previously discovered 'reading circuit' in the brain was activated during letter perception. However this only occurred after handwriting not after tracing or copying that are frequently used in early years education. Their conclusion was that handwriting supported symbol-sound knowledge development in normal subjects. It was a connection made implicitly during contact with print. It suggests that it is a process that occurs normally during literacy teaching by 'Look and Say' methods and can be facilitated by systematic phonics systems leading to lower incidences of dyslexia. It is also the reason why multisensory phonogram training has been incorporated into the more successful remediation regimes. In dyslexics there appears to be a disruption in the neurological system so that very specific and often repetitive training is needed initially to overcome the 'phone' barrier. After this has been done, the whole process speeds up.

Geschwind [34] identified dissociation in dyslexia in the left angular gyrus. This is where sounds and symbols would be connected (by articulatory feel/movements), but in dyslexics this connection appears to be broken. It therefore needs to be restored by overtraining, or other areas of the brain have to be taught to take over the 'pickup' function. This is most possible in the youngest brains. Using in-air tracing of the letters then writing them free-form on the paper, the Fernald [35] method, and using MAPT and cursive or joined writing, based upon practices in the specialist dyslexia, alphabetic-phonic-syllabic-linguistic (APSL) programmes were part of the intervention system.

In 2012 four primary schools were recruited to take part in a pilot project. Each school had one to three Foundation (Reception year) classes, eight classes in all (N = 175). The children were just 5 years old and a few were 'rising fives'. Their eight teachers were asked to collect one piece of copy writing and one piece of completely unaided (free-form) writing after the children had been 1 month in the school. The month was to allow them to settle into the school routines. The two writing samples were to be written on separate days using the materials they were now used to using in their class. For example, most would be telling their 'news' and then copy writing it. Some teachers would give them lines to write on, others would not and all the subjects would be using pencils. The free-form writing would be less common, and so the teachers' learning managers were the intermediaries who would ensure the rules were kept.

The teachers were told they would receive a report on the progress of each child from the marks they had made on the two pieces of work and also what might be done to help them progress. The first results were collected in October, and a second set of free-form writing was collected in March 2013 in the following year to check on any progress that had been made by the children. The reports were sent to schools in January and late May (2013). Schools A and B were in the disadvantaged areas and schools C and D in the advantaged areas (**Table 2**).

As can be seen, the children in the advantaged areas entered school with better writing skills than those in the less advantaged areas. This is not an unexpected result. In research for the Sutton Trust, Jerrim [36] found that children from disadvantaged backgrounds by the end of the Reception year were 5 months behind peers in reading development. It was significant that once they fell behind, they remained behind and failed to catch up later, and they were already consigned to underachieve by 6 years old. The tendency has been for teachers to regard a lack of writing skills in these early years as non-problematic [37] because the children will 'catch up' given more time to mature and activities to develop the necessary skills. However the research indicates that this is most unlikely.

The free-form writing scores were marked on a 10-point rating scale for 'spelling'. The spelling scale was established by scrutinising all 175 scripts in the F1 cohort and placing them in a rank order from random marks and scribble through to more or less correct spelling. A similar process was used to develop a handwriting

Class	Nos.	Free writing 1	Free writing 2	Nos. 'at risk'
A1	17	2.33	7.12	3 + 2
A2	18	2.44	4.3	11+
B1	21	3.24	6.13	4 + 2
C1	28	6.11	6.76	0
C2	27	5.37	6.1	5 + 3
Totals	111	4.29	5.32	23 + 7
Borderline nos.: 23 = scored 4				
Private school, initial results (F1)				
D1	21	3.57		
D2	22	3.5		
D3	21	4.05		
Totals	64	3.71		
This school left the project before task F2				
Free writing F1 = October 2012 sample: N = 175 (2 absentees)				
Free writing F2 = March 2013				

Table 2.
Results from the pre- and post-test free-form writing task.

checklist, but clinical items were included [5, 14]. The strategy was to identify the statement that most typifies the writing sample and award that 'score' or rank. A 'score' of 5 was pivotal in that it identified those children who had just 'cracked the alphabetic code'. This is best seen in their attempts to make words using 'skeletal phonics or phones' such as 'wt' for 'went', 'ws' for 'was', 'goig' for 'going' and 'se' for 'she' or single letter sounds to represent a word 'w' for 'was'. Phonetics would be represented by 'kwiz' for 'quiz', 'buk' for 'book', 'apl', 'nite', 'marster', 'berd', 'butiful' and so on.

Correct spelling of common words such as 'I', 'the', 'and' and 'my' did not count as phonic achievement as they are so commonly used in copy writing they can often be recalled visually rather than phonetically. The reports focused upon the explicit teaching of sounds by first feeling the consonants in the mouth and mouthing them and feeling them as they wrote the grapheme—MAPT.

3.1 Ranks for free-form spelling

1. Random marks.

2. Scribble, marks in some order.

3. Marks, mandalas roundels, occasional letters, possibly in lines.

4. Some letter shapes and letters, in a line.

5. Letters, possible phones.

6. Word forms, letters, phone(s) evident (the critical achievement).

7. Some phonic skeletons, word bits and phones, some meaning.

8. Skeletal phonics, phonetics, some words, meaning apparent.

9. Some correct words, phonics, phonetics, meaning mostly clear.

10. More correct spelling, skeletal phonics, meaning clear.

11. Mainly correct spelling, legible, systematic word spaces.

In October 2012 Millie's script in **Figure 4** is firmly written but with some conventional letter forms, but there is no sign that she is using them as phones as yet. She is on the borderline for cracking the alphabetic code; some direct MAPT teaching of M in her name and 'i' and 't' should help her begin.

In October 2012 James's script on entry to Reception *'I took grandad to the lidrary'* scores 9 for spelling. The spelling is almost correct, the meaning is clear, but word spaces are not well defined yet. In comparison with Millie's script, his shows some coordination difficulties. For example, the script is faint, there is variation in pressure and 'wobble and shake' on the letter strokes. The letter bodies vary in size, and some letters are 'drawn' rather made in monoline, e.g. 'g' and 'y'. He scored 7 on the Handwriting checklist.

In March 2013 Bethan's emergent writing scores 8:

'at esd tighm weeget cheoklurt'.

'At Easter time we get chocolate'. This is a very good phonetic and phonic representation of her message and some word spaces this time. Good skill development. However she is not forming some of her letters efficiently so will need some direct teaching of how to make, for example, 'a' 'd' 'g' 't' 'h' with one continuous line instead of two.

3.2 Interobserver reliability

Twenty spelling scripts were selected from the whole pack and were used as training items to teach a naïve assessor how to use the scale so that an interobserver reliability coefficient of the instrument could be calculated. After 30 minutes training using the spelling scale on the 20 illustrative scripts, the naïve assessor was given all 111 scripts from schools A, B and C to assign a rank out of 10. The coefficient of agreement with the experimenter was +0.81. It was +0.93 when a small number of differences of one scale point were exempted. When the experimenter remarked the scripts after a delay of 1 month, the coefficient of agreement between assessments was +0.98. This showed that the categories were stable, and later a sample of experienced Reception teachers at two conferences were able to use them effectively and found the scale useful.

Girls consistently outperformed boys in each of the schools and classrooms.

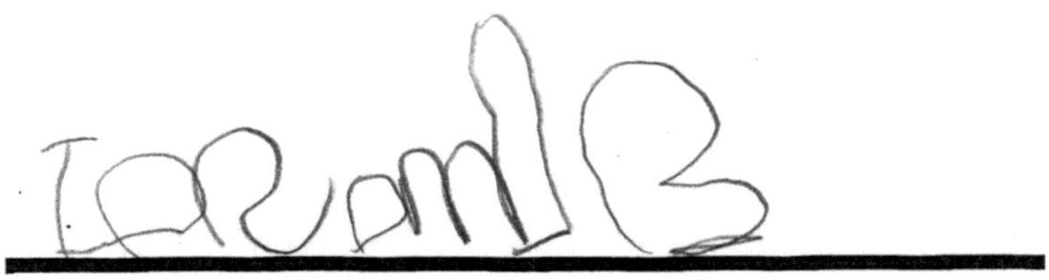

Figure 4.
Millie. I went to nanny's: Scores 4.

	Boys	Girls	N
A + B social housing	2.38	3.03	56
C owner occupier	4.52	6.81	55
D private school	3.34	4.06	64
	3.51	4.41	175

Table 3.
Initial socio-economic advantages in spelling scores.

The scores in **Table 3** show that school C children consistently obtained higher scores than the other two schools in the same local area and confirmed the disadvantages associated with being poor that were found for reading by Jerrim [36].

In **Table 3**, the ratio of 'at risk' boys to girls was 1.4–1 and not the standard 4–1 [4]. This was 27% of the cohort after 5 months in school that had not broken the 'phone' barrier. By the end of a further term in Reception, it would be likely that others would do this leaving about 20% at risk on entry to Year 1. The whole one third however would be unlikely to catch up with peers throughout their school careers according to Jerrim [36] in the Sutton Trust Research. These three schools were the feeder schools to a local state secondary school with a comprehensive entry.

In a Year 7 writing research project with this school [38], 18.6% of the cohort had spelling difficulties that put them in the 'dyslexia zone', and one third had poor spelling. This meant that they were failing the HMCI [39] criterion making more than 5 misspellings per 100 words. Although these researches were cross-sectional rather than longitudinal, the failing group sizes were remarkably similar, e.g. approximately 20% in the dyslexic zone and one third of the cohorts in the disadvantaged group at Reception and in Year 7. The dyslexic zone at the secondary school stage may seem large, but it included those who are often called 'hidden' dyslexics with spelling but not reading problems (dysorthographics).

4. Diagnostic and remediation interventions in the research

Data on 'early marks' on paper had been collected over a number of years on visits to Reception classes for teaching supervision, appraisal and reading research. As a result a pilot study in a London school was set up in 1997–1998. The school was in 'special measures' and requested appraisal help. It was found that the reading teaching method was entirely 'Look and Say' and the disadvantaged backgrounds from which the children came offered little literacy support. In order to redress the balance, a programme was written for them introducing MAPT, and a teaching progression developed from the remedial TRTS [15] system. This was based on the Hickey Multisensory Language Programme [40] that was in itself an anglicised version of the Gllingham and Stillman [41] programme—the 'Red Book' edition.

This specialist programme would teach MAPT and word building from the outset and cursive writing. The programme was called *Developmental Spelling* [20]. The pilot study was carried out in the school, which was already teaching cursive writing. The school SATs results for 1997 and then 1998 after using the programme intervention gave the following results (**Table 4**).

The maths scores show the potential of the children and some good teaching, whereas the literacy scores show a need for some serious intervention. Although the MAPT programme was devoted to spelling and achieved approximately 30% uplift, it can also be seen to transfer to reading and give reading support with 10% uplift.

	1997	1998
Reading	46%	56%
Spelling	16%	44%
Writing	57%	58%
Maths	83%	85%

Table 4.
SATs results for the FLane school.

Remedial programmes that did not give sustained attention to spelling were found not to be able to give the 2-year uplift that was required [1, 26].

In the interim a series of government initiatives took place such as the National Literacy Strategy (NLS, 1998) that failed and then Phonics First [11], which seemed not to have the impact that had been expected. As a result any independent research intervention in schools was not possible in that period except for some research projects by our MA students in independent schools. Their casework with dyslexics identified as falling behind in Reception even after the structured support found that they usually had both dysgraphia and dyslexia—more complex needs. In their cases daily individual tuition using the reading and spelling packs from Hickey MLC or TRTS for the first five letters brought the pupil up to the level of peers [42]. Other pupils with less severe difficulties were found to be able to move forward with the Developmental Spelling programme alone and their normal class reading teaching methods.

Free writing of news as in the above examples, sometimes called 'free-form', 'emergent' writing or 'creative spelling' [10] has the advantage over reading in that the evidence it provides is concrete and records the child's developing knowledge. Although handwriting has been given little attention in English education in recent years [43], it also appears to play a more important role in reading development than has hitherto been understood as found in research with preliterate children by James and Engelhardt [33].

They found that the initial duplication process mattered a great deal. When children had drawn a letter freehand, they exhibited increased activity in three areas of the brain that were activated in adults when they read and write. These were the left fusiform gyrus, the inferior frontal gyrus and the posterior parietal cortex. It showed that handwriting supports sound-symbol knowledge development and provides another reason for using the MAPT training technique during the early learning of letters and their sounds. Solity [44] found that children only needed to learn a handful of sound-symbol associations to start them on their literacy learning. This is why it is essential to give them the training on /i/t/p/n/s/ because they can be used to build 25 words.

A writing component in dyslexia remediation is also endorsed by studies that showed spelling acquisition was greater when accompanied by writing activities as opposed to reading alone [45, 46]. Remediation programmes such as the Hickey Multisensory Language Course (HMLC) failed to give a 2-year uplift in each year when the spelling pack work and dictations were omitted [47]. In relation to later achievement, Berninger [48] found that the two best predictors of good composition in the later years were speed in writing the letters of the alphabet and coding them (writing the symbols for the letter sounds).

The present research had begun in 2012 when state schoolteachers seemed to become ready again to try new literacy initiatives. In this research having established the nature of the spelling/writing difficulties in the 175 scripts, a rank order of spelling skills was developed. Each script was analysed for the level of spelling skill in relation to the scale as well as handwriting competence. A scale point of 5 was identified as critical in that it showed that the child had correctly just linked a sound with its symbol and used it in writing, and it was termed a 'phone' to distinguish it. It showed that a child had just begun to 'crack the alphabetic code' [49]. If this was the case, then profiles of dyslexic development showed that he or she was unlikely to become dyslexic. What was also found to be critical in dyslexics' progress was to build words, and this needed to be done from the outset of the programmes.

This new research offered an opportunity to test the effectiveness of the interventions using MAPT and word building with Reception (Foundation) Year and Year 1 children. In this cohort of over 100 children from a coastal area in England, it would be predicted that 10 of them would become dyslexic and at least 4 of them would have severe dyslexia and would not be able to write legible, readable messages by the time they were 7 years old, the traditional time when they might be identified. In this area it had been found that one third of their feeder secondary school pupils had significant difficulties with spelling and 18.6% were in the dyslexic category making more than 10 different errors per 100 words [38].

The eight teachers were sent a copy the *Developmental Spelling Handbook* as well as the reports on each of their pupils as for Hana and Freddie below. They contained a diagnosis of motor and spelling skill with suggestions on how the skills could be improved. The 111 reports were sent to the schools' learning managers in February 2013, late May 2013 and again in December 2014. The teachers could choose whether or not to implement any of the ideas, and some seemed more proactive than others in this respect especially the teacher of class A1. The results are shown in **Table 2**. The teachers in Year 1 could also choose to follow up on the programme based on the reports the results follow.

5. The follow-up study 2014

Two years later, in September 2014, the three State schools left in the project provided another sample of their pupil's writing on entry into Year 2. This time it was a 10-minute free writing 'test' on a favourite topic of the child's choice. They were given a few minutes to think and plan what they would write. Two schools A and C now responded (N = 93 pairs of scripts). There were 4 Year 2 classes altogether, 2 classes with 35 subjects from School A and 58 subjects from School C who had participated in the original Reception year study. The hypothesis was that if the teachers had been influenced by the reports and implemented some of the suggestions, instead of there being 10 dyslexics per 100 subjects, there might be just 1 or 2 per 100 subjects. Example profiles of two typical sets of reports are shown below for Georgia and Freddie.

Georgia: October 2012 copy writing (5): Copies all the words, good-sized writing cannot fit it all in quite. Uses capital A's and reverses form of 'y's. Brofeo for 'brother' indicates use of a phone so may have more in her repertoire if this can be explored. May just have cracked the code although emergent writing does not show this. Has two of the letters in her name 'G' and 'A' and some letter-like forms.

Emergent writing (3): Makes letters 'e' and 'o' as letter shapes. Has not 'cracked the code' here yet. Suggests focus upon teaching the two easy letters and their sounds and names such as 'i' and 't' and shows how words can be built using them, adding 'e' and 'o' soon to help with writing her name.

Emergent writing b. March 2013 (9): 'I think it is kuld in spias'. The meaning is very clear. There are word spaces, and she is using whole word knowledge plus good phonic skills. This suggests she has a good visual memory as well as phonic ability. Good clear writing of a reasonable size, suggest encourage joining now.

October 2014 Year 2 free writing: Georgia wrote 112 words 11.2 w.p.m. above average for the year group and made 7 misspellings 6.25%. No coordination difficulties noted.

Freddie: October 2012 copy writing (1): Traces over the yellow letters with variation in pressure and some wobble. Nearly manages to copy 'I went', but it deteriorates to a very shaky and faint 'w' and an 'e' upside down followed by 't' then 't' in 'to' and ends there (I went to the hospital). Shows coordination difficulties, so will need strengthening, rhythm and pattern training to support the writing skill.

Emergent writing a (2): Makes one or two very large letters (F) and letter shapes in a line. Has not 'cracked the code' but did appear to understand the writing task.

March 2013 emergent writing b. (2–3): He makes some very large letter shapes (half a page long) that include 'i', 'F' and possibly 'n'. The marks are shaky but clear and in a line showing some development of motor skill and writing knowledge. However coordination difficulties are still apparent, and he needs some direct teaching to help him develop some basic phonic knowledge beginning with 'onsets' in reading and 'I spy' games.

His message is 'Daddy, granddad, Nana, mummy, Keith, Joshy, Benben, Leo – we all went on a holiday and took a picnic'. There is a sense of desperation here in that his message is long, coherent and interesting, but his writing skills do not match it. This mismatch makes him a candidate for dyslexia if he cannot 'crack the code' soon. Try articulatory phonics with onsets.

October 2014: Year 2: Wrote 52 words, 5.2 w.p.m., and made 14 misspellings—25.93%.

Coordination difficulties noted in (a) and (b). Writing speed is significantly below average for this age group. It should be seven to eight words per minute. Spelling is in the dyslexic range but mainly likely to be because of the delays caused by his coordination difficulties.

Ninety-three matched pairs of scripts were identified and analysed. The overall totals for the two schools on entry to Year 2 are as follows:

- Mean writing speed was 6.91 words per minute
- Mean spelling error rate was 12.9 per script

Mean writing speeds of students in schools were found to be 1 word more than their chronological age [5, 50]. The results in **Table 5** show that the disadvantaged groups were writing more slowly than the mean for their age group and the advantaged groups were writing faster. This is one more reason why the disadvantaged groups will be prone to underachieve in school and university [48].

To test the predictive value of the spelling scale, the scores were added together for F1 and F2 emergent writing and tested against the spelling error scores of the same pupils in Year 2, as well as their words per minute; the Spearman's rho

	Nos.	w.p.m.	Sp errors	Sp err %
		Means	Means	
School A1	18	5.57	13.41	22.4%
School A2	17	5.66	14.34	25.7%
Totals	35	5.61	13.88	24.0%
School C1	33	7.93	14.61	18.26%
School C2	25	7.76	9.28	12.67%
Totals	58	7.86	12.31	15.47%

Table 5.
Writing speed and spelling results from year 2 (N = 93).

correlations were significant at the $p < 0.01$ level for free-form writing and spelling (+0.58) and (+0.51) accounting for 29 and 25% of the variance. The correlations between words per minute and early spelling skills were not significant except for Class C2 (+0.48). This suggested an approach to teaching writing that valued correct spelling over encouraging developmental spelling. Or it was possibly an idea held by the children that it was more important to get things right than to learn from error. This may well be a disadvantaging approach in years to come in problem solving contexts. It may also be a consequence of lower social status rearing techniques as well as teacher attitude.

At the end of Year 2, the schools taking part in the Writing Research Project were entered for the national SATs, and the results are shown in **Table 6**. In 2015 the 2014 SATs results from the three local schools were collected from the Government Website.

The percentages are of children reaching Level 2 at Key stage 1 in the three schools. The project children in all three schools showed significant improvements in their results compared with the three previous years. The literacy improvements in the low socio-economic status schools (SES) A and B were in the region of 30% and 10% in the already high scores of the advantaged school C. It suggests that the teachers in these schools had implemented some of the techniques and this had benefited the children through the end of the Reception year and into Year 1. SATs results of other schools in the area did not show significant uplifts such as these.

After 19 months the main factors affecting the cohort's achievements were residual coordination difficulties, legibility and orthographic spelling problems. The analysis of the scripts also revealed some factors about the current teaching methods in the schools. It showed that 'Phonics First' and synthetic phonics were not much in evidence. Guided letter formation and the use of lines to write on would be prominent in a list of advisory points as well as removing tracing and copying from the schools' agenda. Of all the scripts from the Year 2 classes, only one was the least decipherable and contained the most primitive spelling. It is typical of spelling seen in the scripts of older or recovering dyslexics entering the alphabetic phase.

In this cohort it was expected that at least 10% would show dyslexic spelling difficulties by the time they reached Year 3 and at least one would be a non-reader and writer like Steven in **Figure 2** above, but this has not proven to be the case, and it is proposed that it was the early attention to 'phones' and word building that helped prevent this. However there was one boy who had handwriting and spelling problems in the alphabetic dyslexic phase.

He wrote at a speed of 4.9 words per minute, which is significantly slower than for the Year 2 age group as a whole (e.g. 7–8 w.p.m.). The script was faint and variable in pressure indicating coordination difficulties. His spelling showed he had cracked the alphabetic code later than other pupils and was just beginning to use it to communicate his ideas. He needed systematic direct teaching of word building using the basic sounds i/t/p/n/s and following the rest of the Developmental Programme.

	2011	2012	2013	2014	2014		
					Reading	Writing	Maths
School A	35%	47%	48%	78%	85%	80%	66%
School B	37%	37%	50%	66%	76%	78%	46%
School C	77%	87%	88%	96%	95%	98%	96%

Table 6.
Key stage 1 SATs results for the three project schools.

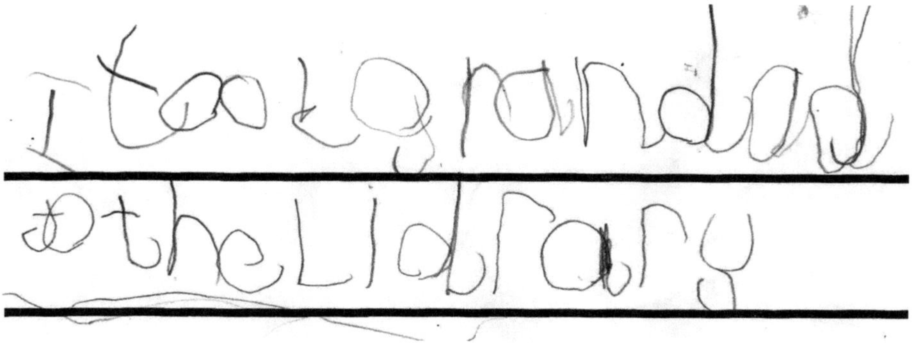

Figure 5.
James. I took granddad to the library: Scores 9.

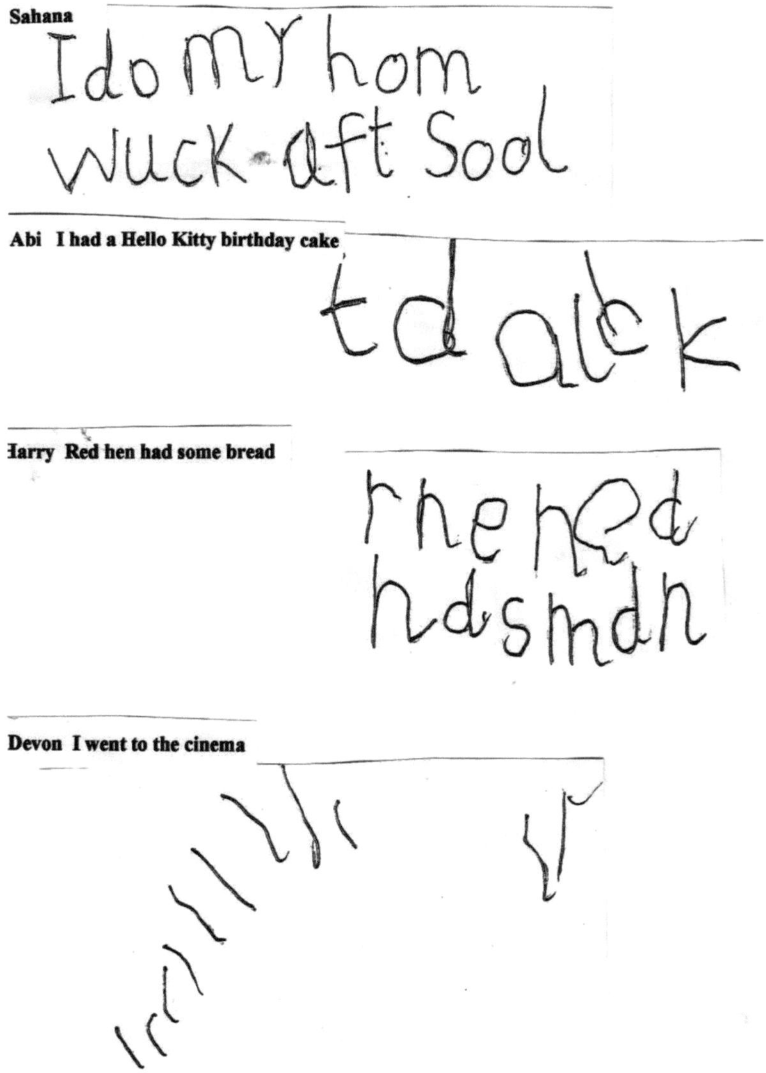
Sahana
Abi I had a Hello Kitty birthday cake
Harry Red hen had some bread
Devon I went to the cinema

Figure 6.
Examples of the range of skills on entry to reception.

Since these pilot studies were completed, funded research in other countries has emerged that supports the underlying principles. For example, Suggate et al. [51] tested 144 German preschoolers (kindergartners) age 6.1 years before reading instruction took place. They were tested on a wide range of cognitive and skills items including fine motor skills (FMS); graphomotor skill, a Greek letter copying task; and writing—they wrote their names and were read 7 letter names to write, and literacy was tested.

They found that the best predictor of decoding (reading) was the ability to copy letters. The study showed that children who could write not only could read better but that early reading went hand in hand with writing. In an earlier study [52], writing letters was shown to be more effective in literacy acquisition than pointing at letters, confirming that implicit transfer from reading to spelling is lower than from spelling to reading.

Ehri's [17] research showed that when there is a basic phonetic structure, children begin to map correct spellings onto this, and this can be seen happening in various scripts in **Figures 4–6**. It shows how important reading is to spelling and writing is to reading and that it is unwise to use only one teaching method especially in the early stages. The 'Phonics First' approach when teachers might try to teach all the sounds before they teach word building or rush pupils on over the phonics ground before they have broken the code is to disadvantage them. Equally delaying the use of Look and Say for reading can also be disadvantageous.

6. Conclusion

In this research how to identify dyslexia in young children a few weeks after their entry to school was shown. It involved discovering if they had understood and could use the alphabetic principle and then giving specific training to those who had not. Pilot studies had shown that this could be effective, and the results in this study confirmed this. Later school SATs showed that the schools in the disadvantaged areas had undergone an uplift of 30% in literacy over previous years as a result of the intervention. In literacy learning pupils will proceed at different rates and steps, and stages will become blurred. It makes research into literacy acquisition through the single lens of reading impossible for resolving the dyslexia problem. What cannot be ignored is the role of implicit learning in literacy [53, 54] and for teachers to take account of this when children arrive at school in order to build upon the knowledge. The free-form writing task enabled this to take place.

The design and use of a spelling rating scale enabled the targeting of teachers' attention to developing 'phones' for use by particular children in both reading and writing. The use of 'phones' or lack of 'phones' in the children's scripts enabled the teachers to intervene and promote them. The intervention strategy was MAPT to overcome any barrier that might be preventing some of the children from easily acquiring alphabetic knowledge. The strategy also identified the severe dyslexic who should have been put on a specialist programme, preferably in the last term in Reception.

The reason that this study is significant is that not only does it identify the literacy of dyslexic and disadvantaged children but that it shows an intervention that can help them overcome their problems. What needs to be investigated thereafter is that if freed from the deficit at an early stage, their literacy can develop normally as teens and adults.

What is now needed is funded research that can train teachers in the technique. This would involve a 2-hour training workshop and then the implementation monitored and the children followed through the elementary school years to evaluate the system in a large replication study. It is expected that this could be extremely cost-effective in human and financial terms both in the short and long term and help overcome the most common learning disability—dyslexia.

Author details

Diane Montgomery
Middlesex University, London, UK

*Address all correspondence to: dmont507@aol.com

References

[1] Montgomery D. Spelling, Handwriting and Dyslexia. London: Routledge; 2007

[2] Al-Hroub A. Types of Developmental Dyslexia in the Arabic Language. Keynote Presentation at the LEAPS Conference on Learning Disabilities. Lebanon: American University of Beirut; 2016

[3] Gelb IJ. A Study of Writing. 2nd ed. London: University of Chicago Press; 1963

[4] BDA. 2019. Available from: www.bda-dyslexia.org.uk. [Accessed: 28 October 2019]

[5] Montgomery D. Dyslexia-Friendly Approaches to Reading, Spelling and Handwriting: A Toolkit for Teachers. London: Routledge; 2017a

[6] Chall J. Learning to Read: The Great Debate. New York: McGraw-Hill; 1967

[7] Chall J. Stages in Reading Development. New York: McGraw-Hill; 1985

[8] Clark MM. Reading Difficulties in Schools. Harmondsworth: Penguin; 1970

[9] Ferreiro E, Teberosky A. Literacy before Schooling. Exeter NH: Heinemann; 1982

[10] Read C. Children's Creative Spelling. London: Routledge and Kegan-Paul; 1986

[11] Rose J. Rose Review. Independent Review of the Teaching of Early Reading: Final Report. London: DfES; 2006

[12] Chomsky C. Write first, read later. Childhood Education. 1971;**47**(6):296-299

[13] Clay MM. What Did I Write? The Beginnings of Reading Development. London: Heinemann; 1975

[14] Montgomery D. Identifying and remediating dyslexia in the reception year. A new possibility? Support for Learning. 2017b;**31**(1):69-80

[15] Cowdery LL, McMahon J, Monrgomery D, Morse P, Prince-Bruce M. Teaching Reading through Spelling. Vol. 2B. Wrexham: TRTS Publishing; 1994

[16] Ehri L, Frith U, editors. Cognitive Processes in Spelling. Chichester: Wiley; 1980

[17] Ehri LC. Acquisition of sight-word reading, spelling memory and vocabulary learning. The role of orthographic mapping. In: Keynote Lecture 11th International Conference of the BDA; April; Telford, UK. 2018

[18] Monroe M. Children Who cannot Read. Chicago: Chicago University Press; 1932

[19] Montgomery D. Spelling: Remedial Strategies. London: Cassell; 1997a

[20] Montgomery D. Developmental Spelling Handbook Maldon: Learning Difficulties Research Project. 1997b. Available from: www.ldrp.org.uk

[21] Brown GDA, Ellis NC, editors. Handbook of Spelling: Theory, Practice and Intervention. Chichester: Wiley; 1994

[22] Snowling MJ. Dyslexia. 2nd ed. Oxford: Blackwell; 2000

[23] Vellutino FR. Dyslexia: Theory and Research. London: MIT Press; 1979

[24] Vellutino FR, Fletcher J, Snowling M, Scanlon D. Specific reading disability (dyslexia) what have we

learned in the past four decades? Journal of Child Psychology and Psychiatry. 2004;**45**(1):2-40

[25] Frith U. Beneath the surface of developmental dyslexia. In: Patterson KE, Marshall JC, Coltheart M, editors. Surface Dyslexia. London: Routledge and Kegan-Paul; 1985

[26] Montgomery D. The contribution of handwriting and spelling remediation to overcoming dyslexia. In: Wydell NT, Fern-Pollak L, editors. Dyslexia—A Comprehensive and International Approach. Rijeka, Croatia: InTech; 2012

[27] Goldberg HK, Shiffman G. Dyslexia. Problems of Reading Disabilities, London: Grune and Stratton; 1972

[28] DfE. National Curriculum, Key Stages 1 and 2. Framework for English and Mathematics. London: DfE; 2014

[29] Gentry JR. Learning to spell developmentally. The Reading Teacher. 1981;**34**(4):378-381

[30] Liberman IY. Segmentation of the spoken word and reading acquisition. Bulletin of the Orton Society. 1973;**23**:365-377

[31] Bryant PE, Bradley L. Children's Reading Difficulties. Oxford: Blackwell; 1985

[32] Bourassa D, Treiman R. Spelling in children with dyslexia: Analyses from the Treiman-Bourassa early spelling test. Scientific Studies of Reading. 2003;**7**(4):309-333

[33] James K, Engelhardt L. The effects of handwriting experience on functional brain development. Neuroscience and Education. 2012;**1**(1):32-42

[34] Geschwind N. Specialisations of the human brain. Scientific American. 1979;**231**(3):156-167

[35] Fernald GM. Remedial Techniques in Basic School Subjects. New York: McGraw-Hill; 1943

[36] Jerrim J. The Reading Gap. Millbank, London: The Sutton Trust; 2013

[37] Whitehead MR. Language and Literacy in the Early Years. 3rd ed. London: Sage; 2004

[38] Montgomery D. Cohort analysis of writing in year 7 after 2, 4, and 7 years of the National Literacy Strategy. Support for Learning. 2008;**23**(1):3-11

[39] HMCI. The Annual Report of the Chief Inspector for Schools in England. London: The Stationery Office; 2001

[40] Augur J, Briggs S, editors. The Hickey Multisensory Language Course. 2nd ed. London: Whurr/Wiley-Blackwell; 1991

[41] Gllingham AM, Stillman BU. Remedial Training for Children with Specific Disability in Reading, Spelling and Penmanship. Bath: Basic Books; 1956

[42] Vallence C. An investigation into the design of a multisensory reading, spelling and handwriting curriculum in a small independent primary school [MA SpLD thesis]. London: Middlesex University; 2008

[43] Medwell J, Strand S, Wray D. What should we assess in primary writing? Handwriting Today. 2008;**7**:23-28

[44] Solity J. Systematic Synthetic Phonics. A Possible Cause of Pupils' Literacy Difficulties. Lecture 11th International Conference of the BDA; April; Telford, UK, 2018

[45] Bosse M-L, Chaves N, Valdois S. Lexical orthography acquisition: Is handwriting better than spelling aloud? Frontiers in Psychology. 2014;**5**. DOI: 10.3389/fpsyg.2014.00056

[46] Ouellette G, Beers A. A not-so-simple view of reading: How oral vocabulary and visual-word recognition complicate the story. Reading and Writing. 2010;**23**(2):189-208. DOI: 10.1007/s11145-008-9159-1

[47] Ridehalgh N. A comparison of remediation programmes and an analysis of their effectiveness in a sample of pupils diagnosed as dyslexic' [MA SpLD Dissertation]. London: Middlesex University; 1999

[48] Berninger VW. Writing problems in developmental dyslexia. Under-recognised and under-treated. Journal of School Psychology. 2008;**46**:1-21

[49] Montgomery D. Teaching pre-reading through training in pattern recognition. The Reading Teacher. 1977;**30**(6):216-225

[50] Allcock P. The importance of handwriting skills in key stage 3 and GCSE examinations of more able pupils. Educating Abled Children. 2001;**5**(1):23-25

[51] Suggate S, Pufke E, Stoeger H. 'Do fine motor skills contribute to early reading development?' Journal of Research in Reading. 2016b Vol. 00, No. 00, 1-19 DOI:10.1111/1467-9817.12081

[52] Suggate S, Pufke E, Stoeger H. The effect of fine and grapho-motor skill demands on preschoolers' decoding skill. Journal of Experimental Child Psychology. 2016a;**141**:34-48

[53] van Daal V. A longitudinal study of self-teaching in learning to read and spell. In: Keynote Lecture 11th International Conference of the BDA; Telford, UK; 12-14 April 2018

[54] NLS. The National Literacy Strategy. London: NLS; 1998

Chapter 5

The Heterogeneity of Reading-Related Difficulties in Chinese

Connie Suk-Han Ho, Edmond Hong-Kei Cheung and Jocelyn Ching-Yan Kwok

Abstract

The present chapter reviews cognitive-linguistic skills which are associated with various reading-related difficulties in Chinese. Research findings have showed that rapid naming and orthographic deficits are the unique marker deficits of Chinese developmental dyslexia. However, studies have indicated overlapping and dissociative deficits in dyslexia and spelling difficulties. Findings on dissociation between word reading and spelling difficulties suggest that weaknesses in orthographic processing may specifically cause difficulties in Chinese word spelling. Deficits in rapid naming are more associated with word reading fluency than reading accuracy. Beyond word level processing, there are children who encounter difficulties in reading comprehension even with adequate decoding skills. This group of specific poor comprehenders was found to be weak in some discourse-level skills, like comprehension monitoring and inferencing. Knowledge of these findings will inform us about effective identification of and intervention for children with difficulties in one or a combination of several reading-related difficulties in Chinese.

Keywords: cognitive-linguistic profile, dyslexia, spelling difficulties, reading comprehension difficulties, Chinese

1. Introduction

At least 10% of individuals may encounter disorders in oral and/or written languages, and this may hamper their long-term learning, social and psychological well-being. Since reading and writing are language-based activities, impairments on reading and writing may be rooted in some language difficulties. According to the Simple View of Reading [1, 2], decoding and language comprehension are the two core components of reading comprehension with empirical support in alphabetic (see Florit and Cain's meta-analysis study [3]) and non-alphabetic writing systems like Chinese (e.g., [4, 5]). This framework is also useful for classifying various types of reading difficulties. Dyslexic children are often found mainly to have decoding problems, while poor comprehenders have difficulties in language comprehension (e.g., [6, 7]). There appears to be differential impairments in decoding and comprehension skills in different poor reader groups (e.g., [8, 9]). The present chapter will discuss the heterogeneity of reading-related difficulties in word reading, spelling, and reading comprehension among Chinese readers.

2. Cognitive profiles of reading and spelling difficulties in Chinese

2.1 Developmental dyslexia: decoding difficulties in Chinese

About a century ago, developmental dyslexia (DD) was called "word blindness," which suggested that for some unknown reasons individuals having this disorder could not recognize words efficiently like people having blindness. Generally speaking, around 3–5% of the school population in a Western country has DD, a severe and persistent difficulty in reading and spelling, which is not a result of any apparent intrinsic or extrinsic causes. Research findings have informed us that DD is a specific genetic language-based disorder and at-risk children may have difficulties learning the spoken language before they formally learn to read. Although there are genetic-basis and neurological differences in DD, our discussion in the present chapter will mainly focus on the cognitive functioning of individuals with reading difficulties.

For people with DD reading an alphabetic writing system, their major cognitive deficits appear to be phonologically based. When reading an opaque language like English, DD readers tend to have weak phonological awareness particularly at phonemic level and in reading nonwords [10–12]. On the other hand, DD readers of more transparent alphabetic systems like Spanish and German, deficit in rapid naming of familiar visual stimuli, instead of phonological awareness, has been found to be a core cognitive deficit (e.g., [12–14]). One possible reason is that with highly regular grapheme-phoneme conversion rules, reading these transparent writing systems does not require strong sensitivity in phonemes as in opaque systems. However, fluent and automatic name retrieval is especially important for reading transparent scripts, especially in reading long words.

There has been an early belief that DD is only a problem for people who speak a Western language (e.g., English, German, and Italian). Early surveys reported a very low incidence of DD among Asian populations (e.g., [15–17]). However, current research findings inform us that children who speak an Asian language (e.g., Chinese, Korean, and Japanese) also have difficulties in reading (e.g., [18–20]). Since Chinese is the major non-alphabetic language with the largest reader population in the world, we would like to understand whether people with DD in Chinese show a cognitive profile different from those reading other alphabetic languages. Before we discuss the cognitive profile of Chinese DD, we will first give a brief account of the Chinese writing system below.

The Chinese writing system is famous for its visually complex orthography. The basic graphic unit in Chinese is a character, and characters are made up of different strokes. In terms of visual complexity, the average number of strokes of 2000 commonly used Chinese characters is 11.2 for the traditional script used in Hong Kong and Taiwan, and 9.0 for the simplified script used in mainland China [21]. Strokes are combined to form stroke-patterns (also called radicals) which may give meaning or sound cues to a character. There are a large number of orthographic units (about 200 semantic radicals and 800 phonetic radicals in Chinese characters [22]) as well as different degrees of positional, semantic, and phonological regularities for these orthographic units.

In terms of phonological structure, Chinese language is special for its monosyllabic nature and its presence of lexical tones, unlike alphabetic languages which are most often multi-syllabic and non-tonal. Each Chinese character is pronounced as a syllable with a fixed grouping of onset, rhyme, and tone. Each Chinese character also represents a morpheme and a much greater proportion of words in Chinese are formed by compounding (e.g., "foot-ball," "basket-ball," "hand-ball," etc.) than in European languages like English. The Chinese writing system is therefore visual-orthographically complex, and more meaning-based than sound-based.

According to the "triangle" model of word reading [23], reading words primarily involves the computation of three types of codes: orthographic, phonological, and semantic. Therefore, orthographic skills, phonological awareness, phonological retrieval, and morphological awareness have been found to be important for word reading both in Chinese and in English [24–28]. It is reasonable to expect that having deficits in these cognitive areas may lead to DD. With the specific characteristics of the Chinese writing system, we would like to identify the cognitive markers which may cause DD in Chinese.

So what constitutes a unique marker deficit for DD? We consider that the marker deficits have to be present only in DD but not in other learning or developmental disorders, for example, specific language impairment or attention-deficit/hyperactivity disorder (ADHD), etc. There may be some common cognitive deficits shared among associated disorders but cognitive deficits unique to DD may better inform us about etiology of the disorder.

Given the orthographic complexity and salience of word compounding morphology in Chinese, orthographic deficits and morphological deficits are expected to be potential candidates of cognitive markers of Chinese DD. Ho and her colleagues have reported that an orthographic deficit and a rapid naming deficit are the major reading-related cognitive deficits in Chinese DD [29, 30]. They have suggested that Chinese dyslexic children show problems in learning orthographic regularities and developing stable and strong orthographic representations that allow rapid retrieval. Although orthographic difficulty may also be found in some English children with dyslexia, this difficulty is more dominant among Chinese dyslexic individuals.

Other studies have shown that morphological awareness is an important predictor of reading success and failure in Chinese (e.g., [31, 32]). For instance, morphological awareness was found to contribute significantly and uniquely to Chinese character reading in kindergarten and grade 2 children, even after controlling for the effects of age, phonological awareness, speeded naming, and vocabulary [27]. Chinese dyslexic children were also found to perform significantly less well than age controls in morpheme production and judgment [32]. Morphological awareness appears to be more important in learning to read Chinese than in learning to read alphabetic languages [31].

To address the issue of unique marker deficits in Chinese DD, we may look into studies which compare the cognitive profile of DD with other learning or developmental disorders. However, this issue was not well examined in past studies. Among the few relevant studies, Ho and her colleagues compared some reading-related cognitive skills in children with different learning or developmental disorders, namely DD, ADHD, developmental coordination disorder (DCD), and borderline intelligence (BI) [33]. They reported that the DD-only group was most impaired in orthographic processing and rapid naming than all other pure groups. They suggested that these two cognitive deficits were unique marker deficits for Chinese DD.

Another study compared some cognitive skills of Chinese first graders with DD, specific language impairments (SLI), and DD + SLI [34]. They reported that orthographic skills and rapid naming were associated with dyslexia; phonological memory and morphological awareness were associated with SLI; and phonological awareness was associated with both. In other studies of lexical tone awareness, both children with DD [35] and children with SLI [36] were found to be weak in tone discrimination and production (a unique phonological feature of the Chinese language). Findings of these studies together appear to show that orthographic deficit and rapid naming deficit are unique marker deficits of DD in Chinese, but morphological or phonological deficit is probably not.

Morphological awareness is first developed in oral language when a child begins to pay attention to how some meaning units (morphemes) can be combined to form different words. Like other oral language skills, morphological awareness may affect development of word reading. However, morphological deficit may be rooted in some language impairments, for example, SLI, instead of a unique cognitive deficit of DD in Chinese. Therefore, difficulty in learning and remembering complicated orthographic patterns and automatic retrieval of arbitrary script-sound associations appear to be unique marker deficits in Chinese DD. This matches well with the characteristics of the Chinese writing system. Since studies on this topic is scarce, more future studies are required to validate this tentative conclusion.

2.2 Dissociation between reading and spelling difficulties in Chinese

Apart from exploring the various marker deficits of DD in Chinese, investigation of manifestations of other reading-related difficulties in Chinese also enhance our understanding of literacy acquisition and difficulties in Chinese. While DD is defined as decoding difficulties (i.e., word reading difficulties), it has an entangled relationship with "encoding" difficulties (i.e., difficulties in spelling). In both research and practice, the concept of "dyslexia" is often conveniently conceptualized as difficulties in both reading and spelling (e.g., [37–39]). Although reading and spelling are highly associated skills, the observed developmental asynchrony of the two skills indicates that they could be non-parallel processes with two partially independent systems [40]. Studies on the dissociation of reading and spelling difficulties have attempted to identify differences between the two systems and provide us with a more comprehensive understanding of reading-related difficulties.

Research has shown that some children experience reading difficulties without having spelling difficulties [41] or vice versa [42]. The prevalence of such dissociated difficulties varies across languages. For Finnish, an orthographically transparent language, it is estimated that 3% of the children have both reading and spelling difficulties (RSD), 1.8% of the children have reading difficulties only (RD), and 2.1% of them have spelling difficulties only (SD). The estimated prevalence rates of RSD, RD, and SD observed in Finnish children are comparable among each other [43]. In contrast, in a study of French users, a relatively less transparent orthography, Fayol et al. [44] have identified a much lower prevalence of RD and SD (both around 4%) as compared with the estimated prevalence of RSD (17.6%). Mixed results were found in studies on languages with high grapheme-to-phoneme consistency (forward regularity) and low phoneme-to-grapheme consistency (backward regularity). Reading is argued to be easier than spelling in these languages because of such asymmetry between forward and backward regularity [45]. As expected, Manolitsis and Georgiou [46] found more SD (8.1%) than RD (5.1%) in their sample of native Greek-speaking children. However, the estimated prevalence rates of SD and RD were comparable in Moll and Landerl's [47] study (SD: 7%; RD: 6.4%) and Wimmer and Mayringer's [41] study (SD: 3.4–5.1%; RD: 4.3–6.4%) with native German-speaking children. Both Greek and German are considered to a high forward regularity (Greek: 95.1%; German: 84%; English as a comparison: 70%) and a relatively lower backward regularity (Greek: 80.3%; German: 47%; English as a comparison: 28%) [41, 46]. Although a larger discrepancy is observed between forward and backward regularity in German, a smaller difference has found between the estimated prevalence rates of SD and RD in German-speaking samples. Such observation does not fully support the hypothesis of Manolitsis and Georgiou [46] that difference in forward and backward regularity has a direct relationship with the resulting prevalence of dissociated difficulties. While the effect of orthographic depth on reading and spelling dissociation is inconclusive, it is evident that much lesser is known about orthographically opaque languages. Under a strict definition, Chinese is not considered as an "opaque orthography" because Chinese is not alphabetic [48]. However, similar to an opaque orthography, Chinese has a very low sound-to-symbol correspondence compared with other languages [49]. The examination of reading and spelling dissociation phenomenon in Chinese complements our understanding of literacy acquisition and difficulties across languages.

The estimated prevalence rates of RSD, RD, and SD among Chinese primary school children are 9.2, 7, and 6.6%, respectively, according to a recent study with a representative sample of Hong Kong grade 4 to grade 6 children [50]. The RSD group was found to perform significantly worse than an age-matched control group of normally achieving children in all the cognitive-linguistic skills measured in the study, including rapid naming speed, phonological memory, morphological awareness, and orthographic skills. All three groups with difficulties were found to perform worse in linguistic comprehension (syntactic skills and discourse skills) when compared with the control group.

The SD group only fell behind the control group in orthographic skills and no significant differences were observed between the two groups on other domains of cognitive-linguistic skills. The SD group also performed the worst on orthographic skills among all four groups in the study. Consistent with past findings, this result supports the essential role of orthographic processing in spelling and impairments in developing efficient orthographic skills and quality orthographic representation may lead to SD. Frith [42] has observed that English-speaking children with SD have a habitual inattentiveness toward words. She has proposed that such inattentiveness may lead to inefficient processing of orthographic information and resulting in an incomplete mental representation of orthographic information, which may be sufficient for reading but not for spelling. Holmes and Quinn [51] have also reported converging evidence indicating inefficient processing of orthographic information in English-speaking individuals with SD. Cheung [52] has replicated Frith's [42] experiment and has found support for both the inefficient orthographic processing hypothesis and the habitual inattentiveness hypothesis in Chinese-speaking children. Consistent with findings from Cheung [50], the SD group in Cheung's [52] study showed no deficits in rapid naming speed or phonological memory. The reported distinctive pattern of deficits of SD highlights a possible independent spelling system in Chinese, which calls for a need for further research on spelling development and difficulties.

The RD only group was found to have difficulties in morphological awareness, phonological memory, and a mild inadequacy in orthographic processing, but not in rapid naming speed [50]. Naming speed deficit is a unique marker deficit for DD in Chinese, it is also consistently found to be present in RD for alphabetic readers [41, 43, 44, 53]. The absence of naming speed deficit in the RD group of Cheung [50] study could partially be explained by differences in measures used in defining the groups. A reading accuracy measure was employed to assess children's reading ability in Cheung's [50] study while the studies on alphabetic readers mentioned earlier used reading fluency measures with/without the addition of reading accuracy measures to assess reading skills of participants because reading accuracy measures are often found to be insensitive in languages with high grapheme-to-phoneme consistency [47]. DD in studies of Chinese is often defined with measures on reading accuracy, reading fluency, and spelling (e.g., [29, 30]).

Cheung's [50] study has also reported another analysis using a combined score of reading accuracy and reading fluency for measuring reading ability. The resulting SD group and the RSD group were found to demonstrate similar characteristics for using reading accuracy score only as the definition. In contrast, the new RD group was found to be slower in naming speed and weaker in morphological awareness when compared with the control group, and the difficulties in phonological memory were no longer observed. The presence of naming speed deficit in the new

RD group but not in the original RD group of this study supports past findings of a stronger association of naming speed with reading fluency but a weaker association with reading accuracy in both alphabetic languages [54] and Chinese [55]. However, it is noteworthy that the participants in Cheung's [50] study are senior graders. Rapid naming, reflecting both paired-associate learning ability and automatic retrieval, may be more associated with word reading accuracy in Chinese junior graders, and with word reading fluency in senior graders.

Conversely, phonological memory deficit was presence in the RD group categorized with reading accuracy measure but not the RD group identified with a combined reading score. Phonological memory is considered to be particularly important in Chinese literacy acquisition because of the emphasis of paired-associate learning in learning Chinese characters [30]. Chinese has a much lower grapheme-to-phoneme correspondence and a much larger pool of distinct graphemes to learn when compared with alphabetic orthographies [49]. Therefore, efficient storage of phonological information would be crucial for learning to read Chinese as the phonological cues from grapheme are relatively ineffective and more associations are needed to be learnt. In Cheung's [52] study on reading and spelling dissociation, he showed that phonological memory has a unique contribution to reading accuracy but not to spelling. These results suggest a unique role of phonological memory on the development of accurate word recognition in Chinese but may play a lesser role in reading fluency and spelling accuracy.

Under both reading assessment conditions of Cheung and colleagues' study, morphological awareness deficit was only found in the RD group and the RSD group but not in the SD group [50]. Morphological awareness was considered to be one of the core cognitive constructs that predict both reading and spelling abilities in Chinese [32, 56]. The absence of morphological awareness deficit in the SD group diverges from our current understanding of the relationship between morphological awareness and spelling development in Chinese. Such a discrepancy indicates a need for further research on the topic.

The distinctiveness between the cognitive profile of RD and SD in Chinese supports the hypothesis of two partially independent systems for reading and spelling. Although there may be some degree of overlap, somewhat different cognitive-linguistic skills are required in acquiring and developing the skills in reading and spelling Chinese words. The non-coinciding profile of deficits of RD and SD reveals the relative importance of morphological awareness and phonological memory on reading and orthographic processing on spelling in Chinese. Naming speed deficit appears to be more associated with word reading fluency than reading accuracy in Chinese. Findings of dissociation studies have enlightened us about the specific roles of some cognitive-linguistic skills on reading and spelling. These conclusions, however, are tentative and further research is required.

2.3 Reading comprehension difficulties in Chinese

Beyond the decoding level, some children experience difficulties in comprehending text. Decoding and reading comprehension processes are inter-related to some extent. Decoding and language comprehension are two important components of reading comprehension as specified by the Simple View of Reading. A number of studies showed that reading comprehension difficulties of children could be attributed to problems in lower order processing, such as word recognition accuracy and speed of word processing although the underlying cognitive processes could be different regarding the types of script of different languages (e.g., [5, 57–59]). In particular, word recognition is more dependent on phonological skill in English than in Chinese as Chinese exhibits a relatively lower word-to-sound correspondence as mentioned earlier [60, 61].

Apart from decoding skill, research in alphabetic languages stressed the importance of language comprehension, defined as "the ability to comprehend spoken language" ([62], p. 369), in reading comprehension. Syntactic awareness, discourse skills, and vocabulary knowledge are the major oral language skills that consistently found to affect reading comprehension even after controlling for word recognition (e.g., [63, 64]). For example, Mokhtari and Thompson [65] examined the relationship of syntactic awareness and reading comprehension performance of fifth graders and found that children's understanding of grammatical structure directly related to reading comprehension performance with a $r = 0.70$ correlation. Another study done by Griffin et al. [66] indicated that oral discourse skills of preschoolers is a significant predictor of reading comprehension performance in later years. In addition to syntactic and discourse skills, vocabulary knowledge is also associated considerably with reading comprehension [67, 68]. Ouellette [68] found that depth of vocabulary knowledge significantly predicted reading comprehension of fourth graders. Furthermore, the amount of receptive and expressive vocabularies a child acquired is linked to decoding proficiency [68].

Research regarding reading comprehension in Chinese suggested that language comprehension skills important for reading comprehension in alphabetic language systems are equally important for Chinese [5, 59, 69]. A model of reading comprehension in Chinese was constructed by Yeung and colleagues [5] through examining the contribution of several reading-related and language comprehension skills, including rapid naming, morphological awareness, verbal working memory, syntactic skills, and discourse skills, to Chinese reading comprehension. Results showed that syntactic and discourse skills predicted Chinese reading comprehension similar to that in alphabetic languages. However, discourse skills measured orally through story-telling and picture arrangement was not as predictive as discourse skills assessed in written format to reading comprehension [5]. One possible reason suggested by the authors was that oral Cantonese and written Chinese were less consistent than many alphabetic languages [5]. Other than syntactic and discourse skills, oral vocabulary was also found to significantly predict reading comprehension of Chinese children. For instance, Chik et al. [69] found that oral vocabulary was a strong predictor of Chinese reading comprehension for children in junior grades although its contribution reduced from senior grades onwards. Altogether, these studies suggested reading comprehension difficulty is not only limited to decoding of scripts but is also highly related to individuals' language comprehension skills no matter in alphabetic languages or Chinese.

Despite the clear links between decoding, language comprehension and reading comprehension, recent research suggested that reading comprehension difficulties could not be merely explained by the decoding efficiency and oral language skills. In fact, researchers found that some children demonstrated adequate decoding skills but still experience difficulties in reading (e.g., [9, 58, 70, 71]). Such word reading and comprehension dissociation have been recently referred to as specific reading comprehension difficulties (S-RCD). In a review done by Landi and Ryherd [72], adolescents with S-RCD displayed weakness in oral language specifically in vocabulary and grammatical processing. Spencer and Wagner [62] conducted a meta-analysis to further investigate the language comprehension skills of children aged 4–12 with reading comprehension difficulties as compared with typical readers. The sample was a mixture of alphabetic and non-alphabetic language speakers with a majority of the data involved English speakers. The results revealed that although the language comprehension skills of children with S-RCD were relatively weak, such weakness could not fully account for the reading comprehension problems, which was found to be more severe than the language comprehension problems [62].

Thus, the specific reading comprehension problems might involve skills beyond the scope of the Simple View of Reading.

Another branch of research investigated the contribution of higher order language skills to reading comprehension which is not theorized in the Simple View of Reading, such as the processing of prosodic information, comprehension monitoring, and inference-making (e.g., [73–79]). For instance, reading comprehension could be impaired if individuals fail to recognize appropriate prosodic features and construct meaningful oral expression [80]. Among the many contributors, comprehension monitoring—an individual's ability to "evaluate his/her understanding of information" [78]—stands out to be uniquely associated with S-RCD. Children with S-RCD was found to be less sensitive to inconsistency and ambiguity in texts than typical readers that they were less able to identify unreasonable information embedded in a passage [73]. Furthermore, they did not display typical slowing in eye movement when encountered ambiguous words in passages as found by an eye-tracking study done by van der Schoot and colleagues [81]. Although some researchers found that individuals with S-RCD exhibit weak inferencing skill—the ability to integrate sentence meaning and make logical deduction—other researchers argued that the inference failure of S-RCD may be more related to the automaticity in integrating information and language comprehension weakness than a deficit in inferencing ability [72, 82]. Thus, the contribution of inferencing skills to S-RCD is yet to be explored.

One important issue to note is that research specifically focused on S-RCD in Chinese is relatively scarce. Zhang et al. [59] attempted to search for the early precursors of reading comprehension difficulties in Chinese children and found that poor comprehenders did not necessarily exhibit word reading deficits, especially later in the development. Thus, they concluded that similar to previous findings on alphabetic language, S-RCD might be present in Chinese but further exploration is needed given some major differences between Chinese and alphabetic languages, such as route of semantic access and processing of grammatical information [59].

To conclude this section, reading comprehension difficulties are multifaceted and heterogeneous in nature. The difference in the manifestations of reading comprehension difficulties could be traced to multiple distinct roots, from word decoding, oral language to higher order language processing, such as comprehension monitoring. Yet, the heterogeneity of reading comprehension difficulties in Chinese remains to be explored in the future.

3. Conclusions

We have reviewed in this chapter the causes and patterns of reading, spelling, and comprehension difficulties in Chinese are heterogeneous. Various research findings together have suggested that rapid naming and orthographic deficits are the unique marker deficits of DD in Chinese. Since DD has been defined by impairments in word reading accuracy, reading fluency, and spelling in Chinese, research on the dissociation between word reading and spelling difficulties has enlightened us about the specific mechanism of word reading and spelling development. Research findings so far suggest that weaknesses in orthographic processing, including inattentiveness to word details, inefficient orthographic processing, and incomplete mental representation of orthographic information, may specifically cause difficulties in word spelling in Chinese. Deficits in automatic name retrieval appear to be more associated with word reading fluency than reading accuracy in Chinese. This is especially true for senior graders who may have learned a basic set of written characters and are beginning to develop automaticity in retrieving the characters for higher level processing, like understanding syntactic relationships and text comprehension. Inefficient word decoding and weak oral language skills (e.g., morphological awareness, vocabulary knowledge, syntactic skills, and discourse skills) have been found to contribute to difficulties in text comprehension. However, some discourse-level skills may contribute to reading comprehension in addition to these two components of the Simple View of Reading. We believe that knowledge about the specific associated cognitive-linguistic skills for word reading, spelling, and text comprehension will inform us how to effectively identify children early with various reading-related difficulties and design timely and appropriate intervention for each specific group.

Acknowledgements

Preparation of this book chapter was supported by the Eugene Chuang Professorship in Developmental and Educational Psychology of the University of Hong Kong, General Research Fund (#17614517), and the Collaborative Research Fund (C4054-17W) of the Hong Kong Special Administrative Region Research Grants Council.

Author details

Connie Suk-Han Ho*, Edmond Hong-Kei Cheung and Jocelyn Ching-Yan Kwok
The University of Hong Kong, Hong Kong, China

*Address all correspondence to: shhoc@hku.hk

References

[1] Gough PB, Tunmer WE. Decoding, reading, and reading disability. Remedial and Special Education. 1986;**7**(1):6-10

[2] Hoover WA, Gough PB. The simple view of reading. Reading and Writing. 1990;**2**(2):127-160

[3] Florit E, Cain K. The simple view of reading: Is it valid for different types of alphabetic orthographies? Educational Psychology Review. 2011;**23**(4):553-576

[4] Ho CS-H et al. Examining an extended simple view of reading in Chinese: The role of naming efficiency for reading comprehension. Contemporary Educational Psychology. 2017;**51**(Supplement C):293-302

[5] Yeung P-s et al. A model of reading comprehension in Chinese elementary school children. Learning and Individual Differences. 2013;**25**:55-66

[6] Catts HW, Hogan TP, Fey ME. Subgrouping poor readers on the basis of individual differences in reading-related abilities. Journal of Learning Disabilities. 2003;**36**(2):151-164

[7] Nation K, Norbury CF. Why reading comprehension fails: Insights from developmental disorders. Topics in Language Disorders. 2005;**25**(1):21-32

[8] Leach JM, Scarborough HS, Rescorla L. Late-emerging reading disabilities. Journal of Educational Psychology. 2003;**95**(2):211-224

[9] Oakhill JV, Cain K, Bryant PE. The dissociation of word reading and text comprehension: Evidence from component skills. Language & Cognitive Processes. 2003;**18**(4):443-468

[10] Frith U. Brain, mind and behaviour in dyslexiain Dyslexia, Biology. In: Hulme C, Snowling MJ, editors. Cognition and Intervention. Singular Publishing Group; 1997. p. 1-20

[11] Snowling MJ. From language to reading and dyslexia1. Dyslexia. 2001;**7**(1):37-46

[12] Ziegler JC, Goswami U. Reading acquisition, developmental dyslexia, and skilled reading across languages: A psycholinguistic grain size theory. Psychological Bulletin. 2005;**131**(1):3

[13] Landerl K et al. Predictors of developmental dyslexia in European orthographies with varying complexity. Journal of Child Psychology and Psychiatry. 2013;**54**(6):686-694

[14] Ziegler JC et al. Developmental dyslexia in different languages: Language-specific or universal? Journal of Experimental Child Psychology. 2003;**86**(3):169-193

[15] Kline CL. Orton-Gillingham methodology: Where have all of the researchers gone? Bulletin of the Orton Society. 1977;**27**(1):82-87

[16] Kuo WF. Assessing and identifying the development and educational needs of the exceptional individual. In: Paper Presented at the World Congress on Future Special Education, Stirling, Scotland; 1978

[17] Makita K. Reading disability and the writing system. In: Merritt JE, editor. New Horizons in Reading. Newark, Delaware: IRA Press; 1974. pp. 250-254

[18] Stevenson HW et al. Reading disabilities: The case of Chinese, Japanese, and English. Child Development. 1982;**53**(5):1164-1181

[19] Hirose T, Hatta T. Reading disabilities in modern Japanese children.

Journal of Research in Reading. 1988;**11**(2):152-160

[20] Chan DW et al. Prevalence, gender ratio and gender differences in reading-related cognitive abilities among Chinese children with dyslexia in Hong Kong. Educational Studies. 2007;**33**(2):249-265

[21] Chan MY. Statistics on the strokes of present-day Chinese script. Chinese Linguistics. 1982;**1**:299-305

[22] Hoosain R. Psycholinguistic Implications for Linguistic Relativity: A Case Study of Chinese. Hillsdale, NJ: Erlbaum; 1991

[23] Seidenberg MS, McClelland JL. A distributed, developmental model of word recognition and naming. Psychological Review. 1989;**96**(4):523

[24] Bowers PG, Wolf M. Theoretical links among naming speed, precise timing mechanisms and orthographic skill in dyslexia. Reading and Writing. 1993;**5**(1):69-85

[25] Hindson B et al. Assessment and early instruction of preschool children at risk for reading disability. Journal of Educational Psychology. 2005;**97**(4):687

[26] Hultquist AM. Orthographic processing abilities of adolescents with dyslexia. Annals of Dyslexia. 1997;**47**(1):89-114

[27] McBride-Chang C et al. Morphological awareness uniquely predicts young children's Chinese character recognition. Journal of Educational Psychology. 2003;**95**(4):743

[28] Hulme C, Snowling M. Deficits in output phonology: An explanation of reading failure? Cognitive Neuropsychology. 1992;**9**(1):47-72

[29] Ho CS-H et al. The cognitive profile and multiple-deficit hypothesis in Chinese developmental dyslexia. Developmental Psychology. 2002;**38**(4):543-553

[30] Ho CS-H et al. Cognitive profiling and preliminary subtyping in Chinese developmental dyslexia. Cognition. 2004;**91**(1):43-75

[31] McBride-Chang C et al. Changing models across cultures: Associations of phonological awareness and morphological structure awareness with vocabulary and word recognition in second graders from Beijing, Hong Kong, Korea, and the United States. Journal of Experimental Child Psychology. 2005;**92**(2):140-160

[32] Shu H et al. Understanding Chinese developmental dyslexia: Morphological awareness as a core cognitive construct. Journal of Educational Psychology. 2006;**98**(1):122

[33] Ho CS-H et al. Reading-related cognitive deficits in developmental dyslexia, attention-deficit/hyperactivity disorder, and developmental coordination disorder among Chinese children. Reading Research Quarterly. 2005;**40**(3):318-337

[34] Wong AM-Y et al. (Dis)connections between specific language impairment and dyslexia in Chinese. Reading and Writing. 2015;**28**(5):699-719

[35] Li W-S, Ho CS-H. Lexical tone awareness among Chinese children with developmental dyslexia. Journal of Child Language. 2011;**38**(4):793-808

[36] Wong AM-Y, Ciocca V, Yung S. The perception of lexical tone contrasts in Cantonese children with and without specific language impairment (SLI). Journal of Speech, Language, and Hearing Research. 2009;**52**(6):1493-1509

[37] Schulte-Körne G et al. Evidence for linkage of spelling disability to

chromosome 15. American Journal of Human Genetics. 1998;**63**(1):279-282

[38] Kalindi SC et al. Beyond phonological and morphological processing: Pure copying as a marker of dyslexia in Chinese but not poor reading of English. Annals of Dyslexia. 2015;**65**(2):53-68

[39] Gori S, Facoetti A. How the visual aspects can be crucial in reading acquisition: The intriguing case of crowding and developmental dyslexia. Journal of Vision. 2015;**15**(1):8-8

[40] Cossu G, Gugliotta M, Marshall JC. Acquisition of reading and written spelling in a transparent orthography: Two non parallel processes? Reading and Writing. 1995;**7**(1):9-22

[41] Wimmer H, Mayringer H. Dysfluent reading in the absence of spelling difficulties: A specific disability in regular orthographies. Journal of Educational Psychology. 2002;**94**(2):272-277

[42] Frith U. Unexpected spelling problems. Group. 1980;**83**:495-515

[43] Torppa M et al. The precursors of double dissociation between reading and spelling in a transparent orthography. Annals of Dyslexia. 2017;**67**(1):42-62

[44] Fayol M, Zorman M, Lété B. Associations and dissociations in reading and spelling French: Unexpectedly poor and good spellers. British Journal of Educational Psychology. 2009;**2**(6):63-75

[45] Bosman AMT, Van Orden GC. Why spelling is more difficult than reading. In: Perfetti CA, Rieben L, Fayol M, editors. Learning to Spell: Research, Theory, and Practice across Languages. Hillsdale, NJ: Lawrence Erlbaum Associates; 1997. pp. 173-194

[46] Manolitsis G, Georgiou GK. The cognitive profiles of poor readers/good spellers and good readers/poor spellers in a consistent orthography: A retrospective analysis. Preschool and Primary Education. 2015;**3**(2):103

[47] Moll K, Landerl K. Double dissociation between reading and spelling deficits. Scientific Studies of Reading. 2009;**13**(5):359-382

[48] Katz L, Frost R. The reading process is different for different orthographies: The orthographic depth hypothesis. In: Frost R, Katz L, editors. Advances in Psychology. Amsterdam, North-Holland; 1992. pp. 67-84

[49] Fok A, Bellugi U. The acquisition of visual spatial script. In: Kao HSR, van Galen GP, Hoosain R, editors. Advances in Psychology. North-Holland; 1986. pp. 329-355

[50] Cheung EH-K, Ho CS-H, Chan D, Chung KK, Tsang SM, Lee SH, et al. Prevalence of isolated reading and spelling difficulties in Chinese: Differential demand of lexical route in reading and spelling. In preparation

[51] Holmes VM, Quinn L. Unexpectedly poor spelling and phonological-processing skill. Scientific Studies of Reading. 2009;**13**(4):295-317

[52] Cheung EH-k. The Heterogeneity of Reading and Writing Difficulties. Pokfulam, Hong Kong, SAR: Department of Psychology, The University of Hong Kong; 2018

[53] Bar-Kochva I, Amiel M. The relations between reading and spelling: An examination of subtypes of reading disability. Annals of Dyslexia. 2016;**66**(2):219-234

[54] Georgiou GK, Parrila R, Kirby JR. RAN components and reading development from grade 3 to grade

5: What underlies their relationship? Scientific Studies of Reading. 2009;**13**(6):508-534

[55] Xue J et al. The stability of literacy-related cognitive contributions to Chinese character naming and reading fluency. Journal of Psycholinguistic Research. 2013;**42**(5):433-450

[56] Tong X et al. Morphological awareness, orthographic knowledge, and spelling errors: Keys to understanding early Chinese literacy acquisition. Scientific Studies of Reading. 2009;**13**(5):426-452

[57] Chen H-C. How do readers of Chinese process words during reading for comprehension. In: Wang J, Inhoff AW, Chen H-C, editors. Reading Chinese Script: A Cognitive Analysis. Mahwah, NJ: Erlbaum; 1999. pp. 261-274

[58] Nation K, Snowling MJ. Semantic processing and the development of word-recognition skills: Evidence from children with reading comprehension difficulties. Journal of Memory and Language. 1998;**39**(1):85-101

[59] Zhang J et al. Longitudinal correlates of reading comprehension difficulties in Chinese children. Reading and Writing. 2014;**27**(3):481-501

[60] Catts HW, Adlof SM, Weismer SE. Language deficits in poor comprehenders: A case for the simple view of reading. Journal of Speech, Language, and Hearing Research. 2006;**49**(2):278-293

[61] Nation K, Snowling MJ. Beyond phonological skills: Broader language skills contribute to the development of reading. Journal of Research in Reading. 2004;**27**(4):342-356

[62] Spencer M, Wagner RK. The comprehension problems of children with poor reading comprehension despite adequate decoding: A meta-analysis. Review of Educational Research. 2018;**88**(3):366-400

[63] Gaux C, Gombert JE. Implicit and explicit syntactic knowledge and reading in pre-adolescents. British Journal of Developmental Psychology. 1999;**17**(2):169-188

[64] Kendeou P et al. Predicting reading comprehension in early elementary school: The independent contributions of oral language and decoding skills. Journal of Educational Psychology. 2009;**101**(4):765-778

[65] Mokhtari K, Thompson HB. How problems of reading fluency and comprehension are related to difficulties in syntactic awareness skills among fifth graders. Reading Research and Instruction. 2006;**46**(1):73-94

[66] Griffin TM et al. Oral discourse in the preschool years and later literacy skills. First Language. 2004;**24**(2):123-147

[67] Lervåg A, Aukrust VG. Vocabulary knowledge is a critical determinant of the difference in reading comprehension growth between first and second language learners. Journal of Child Psychology and Psychiatry. 2010;**51**(5):612-620

[68] Ouellette GP. What's meaning got to do with it: The role of vocabulary in word reading and reading comprehension. Journal of Educational Psychology. 2006;**98**(3):554-566

[69] Chik PP-m et al. Contribution of discourse and morphosyntax skills to reading comprehension in Chinese dyslexic and typically developing children. Annals of Dyslexia. 2012;**62**(1):1-18

[70] Keenan JM et al. Issues in identifying poor comprehenders. L'Année Psychologique. 2014;**114**(4):753-777

[71] Rønberg LF, Petersen DK. It matters whether reading comprehension is conceptualised as rate or accuracy. Journal of Research in Reading. 2016;**39**(2):209-228

[72] Landi N, Ryherd K. Understanding specific reading comprehension deficit: A review. Lang & Ling Compass. 2017;**11**(2):e12234

[73] Cain K, Oakhill JV. Profiles of children with specific reading comprehension difficulties. British Journal of Educational Psychology. 2006;**76**(4):683-696

[74] Cain K et al. Comprehension skill, inference-making ability, and their relation to knowledge. Memory and Cognition. 2001;**29**(6):850-859

[75] Groen MA, Veenendaal NJ, Verhoeven L. The role of prosody in reading comprehension: Evidence from poor comprehenders. Journal of Research in Reading. 2019;**42**(1):37-57

[76] Han F. Comprehension monitoring in Chinese reading among Chinese adolescent readers. Theory and Practice in Language Studies. 2017;**7**(4):241-247

[77] Ho CS-H, Fong CY-C, Zheng MO. Contributions of vocabulary and discourse-level skills to reading comprehension among Chinese elementary school children. Applied PsychoLinguistics. 2019;**40**(2):323-349

[78] Oakhill JV, Hartt J, Samols D. Levels of comprehension monitoring and working memory in good and poor comprehenders. Reading and Writing. 2005;**18**(7):657-686

[79] Oakhill JV, Cain K. Children's difficulties in text comprehension: Assessing causal issues. The Journal of Deaf Studies and Deaf Education. 2000;**5**(1):51-59

[80] Whalley K, Hansen J. The role of prosodic sensitivity in children's reading development. Journal of Research in Reading. 2006;**29**(3):288-303

[81] van der Schoot M et al. Lexical ambiguity resolution in good and poor comprehenders: An eye fixation and self-paced reading study in primary school children. Journal of Educational Psychology. 2009;**101**(1):21-36

[82] Cain K, Oakhill JV. Inference making ability and its relation to comprehension failure in young children. Reading and Writing. 1999;**11**(5):489-503

Chapter 6

Students with Mathematics Learning Disabilities and Their Ways of Thinking in Fraction Learning

Suprih Widodo and Trisno Ikhwanudin

Abstract

This chapter presents the result of research on ways of thinking of students with mathematics learning disabilities in fraction learning. We conducted a class of fraction learning with Lesh translation model. From the class discussion, interview, and students' work, we then explore the students' ways of thinking when they learn fraction. In the class, students with mathematics learning disabilities perform two mental acts with corresponding ways of thinking and ways of understanding; those are interpreting and problem-solving. We find some interesting findings and they are: (1) students know the common denominator method in the addition of fractions; however, they incorrectly apply the method; (2) students use the common denominator approach (for fraction addition) in the multiplication of fraction; and (3) in the division of fraction, students mistakenly apply the invert multiply algorithm.

Keywords: students with mathematics learning disabilities, fraction learning, ways of thinking

1. Introduction

We may have heard the case of a student having difficulty in mathematics, but the student does not experience obstacles in other subjects in school. After further observation, it turns out that the IQ of the student was at an average level even above average. For cases like this, the student can be suspected of having dyscalculic symptoms or mathematics learning disabilities (MLD). Based on the results of the study, the number of people with MLD according to Strauss is 5–8% of school-age children [1], while according to Adler, the number of people with dyscalculia is 5–6% of all children [2].

Research on dyscalculia is still ongoing. Researchers, especially in the United Kingdom and the United States continue to conduct studies to study dyscalculia in greater depth. Therefore, the understanding and understanding of dyscalculia will continue to develop. The following are some of the dyscalculia definitions issued by both formal institutions and individual researchers. Definition of dyscalculia issued by the National Center for Learning Disabilities is as follows: dyscalculia is a term related to learning difficulties in mathematics. Although learning barriers differ from person to person, the general characteristics are as follows: difficulty in numerating, learning numbers, and doing mathematical calculations; difficulty in measurement, showing time, counting money, and estimating the number; problematic in mathematical intelligence and problem-solving strategies [3].

In general, dyscalculia is an umbrella term used for various difficulties in learning mathematics, such as developmental dyscalculia, mathematical difficulties, difficulty learning numerical concepts, and difficulties about learning number concepts.

There are many studies that discuss MLD students, with a different research focus: first, the research that focuses on the identification or criteria of MLD students; second, the research that focuses on how MLD students think in learning mathematics; and third, the research that focuses on finding solutions to learning mathematics in MLD students. The detailed of the research focus is as follows:

1.1 Research that focuses on the identification or criteria of MLD students

The study of the identification and criteria of MLD students has been carried out by several researchers, including the following: Geary described dyscalculia as a numerical and arithmetic difficulty caused by brain injury; he uses this term to describe a population of 5–8% of school-age children who have a cognitive disorder that affects their ability to learn concepts or procedures in one or more areas of mathematics [4].

Next the opinions of several experts about the criteria of MLD students will be described:

- students with an average IQ whose standardized test scores are below the 20th or 25th percentile [4];
- slower and often make mistakes in processing the representation of numbers, for example, the symbol number "3" and the equivalent of the non-symbol "◆◆◆" [5];
- make mistakes in comparing and estimating numbers [6];
- wrong in doing arithmetic calculations [7]; and
- wrong in solving numbers problems that are very easy, for example, $4 \times 5 = 20$ [8].

The researchers identified students with MLD using standardized test results, for example, the Woodcock-Johnson Test of Achievement and the Wide Range Achievement Test, by looking at students who were below the 20th or 25th percentile [9]. Lewis further tightens the criteria for identifying MLD students, which combines the following three criteria:

- students score below 25th percentile on standardized mathematics tests;
- the results of observations and interviews revealed that there was no influence of environmental or social factors on students' inability in mathematics; and
- after being given treatment, the effect of the treatment on increasing mathematical ability is very less. To find this out, Lewis made a comparison with a control class whose members were not MLD students [10].

In identifying students with MLD, Lewis [9] suggests that if researchers use self-developed identification instruments, it is also necessary to include the results of standardized measuring instruments as a comparison. The next suggestion is to apply a cutoff under the 10th percentile; observing longitudinal data showing that learning difficulties in mathematics are long-standing, and researchers must distinguish the difficulty of learning mathematics is the result of cognitive or non-cognitive factors. To do this it is recommended to conduct a demographic analysis of the respondents, for example, socioeconomic status, ethnicity, and mother tongue. This can also be done with qualitative methods, such as interviews, questionnaires, observation of students, parents, and teachers, to find out the factors that lead to the low mathematical achievement of students.

1.2 Research that focuses on MLD students' way of thinking in learning mathematics

The study of how MLD students think in learning mathematics has been carried out by several researchers, including the following:

Lewis states that students with MLD have a different mindset in understanding fractions, she looked at students with MLD does not mean they have deficiencies in understanding the concept of fractions, but there are differences in the way of thinking in understanding fractions [11]. Then Lewis states that students with MLD experience obstacles in learning fractions, especially on the topic of fraction comparison, both fraction comparisons with the same denominator, as well as in fractions comparisons involving fractions of half; in this study Lewis suggested examining students' understanding of the quantity of fractions [12].

Hunt et al. [13] state that MLD students have obstacles in mastering the concept of fractions by learning part-whole models. Newton et al. [14] state that the main error pattern in understanding fractions in MLD students is the use of traditional algorithms that are wrong.

1.3 Research that focuses on finding solutions for MLD students in learning mathematics

The study of alternative mathematical learning solutions for MLD students has been carried out by several researchers, including the following:

Shin and Bryant state that good fraction teaching by MLD students must involve the following 5 aspects: real objects and visual representations such as pictures and number lines, explicit and systematic learning, various time frames and sets of examples, heuristic strategies, and use real problem [15].

Mazzocco et al. state that visual models can be used as alternatives when helping MLD students understand fractions [16]. Gersten et al. [17] state that in assisting MLD students, practitioners are expected to take the following steps: (a) teach students with diverse teaching examples; (b) directing students to say the thoughts and solutions of a problem; (c) teach students to visualize math problems that they face; (d) teach students with diverse/heuristic strategies; (e) the teacher prepares a partner/discussion partner for MLD students; (f) teach MLD students with explicit instructions; (g) the teacher prepares the correct variety and sequence of examples;

Shin and Bryant [15] state that the use of a computer program, Fun Fraction, can help MLD students solve problem-solving in the form of stories. Virtual manipulation in Fun Fraction helps problem-solving skills because students are assisted by this program in representing the problem stories they are dealing with.

Finally, Tian, Jing, and Siegler, state that the use of an optimal number line model can help MLD students understand fraction size and calculation [18].

In this chapter, we focus on students' ways of thinking in fractions learning. It is needed as an essential first step toward effective instructional methods. We use the theory of mental act, ways of thinking, and ways of understanding from

Harel. Furthermore, we also analyze the error pattern of MLD students when they learn fractions. The results of this study are expected to add to the discourse of educational scholarship, especially on the teaching and learning mathematics in an inclusive setting for students with MLD.

2. Fraction learning

Fractional topics include material in mathematics that is difficult to explain. This is because fraction is one of the topics in mathematics that requires high-level and complex thinking. Definition of fractions according to Clarke et al. [19]:

"Fractions are symbolic-shaped expressions that represent the quotient of two numbers $\frac{a}{b}$(where b is not equal to zero). So all rational numbers expressed in terms $\frac{a}{b}$ are fractions, but rational numbers 1.45 are not fractions. Rasonals 1.45 can be called a fraction if written $\frac{145}{100}$. So that all rational numbers can be written as fractions, but there are some important fractions that are not rational numbers, for example: $\frac{a}{b}$ or $\frac{a}{b}$" (p. 15).

In many classes, fractions are taught only in a procedural way. The teacher usually teaches fractions by applying the method of equalizing the denominator, by calculating the Least Common Multiples (LCM). On the other hand, according to Hiebert and Wearne [20], with this procedural method, students will only gain procedural understanding or syntax thinking. Students will not understand the relationship between fractions, in other words, students' conceptual understanding (semantic thinking) will be weak.

How can students gain a conceptual understanding of fractional material? Riccomini suggests two teaching strategies for better fraction learning; the two strategies are learning fractions by using number lines and the use of diverse representations [21]. The use of number lines and paper folding as representations is also suggested by Wyberg et al. [22].

Several other research results also support the use of diverse representations. Dey and Dey suggest the use of geometry representations; addition, subtraction, multiplication, and division operations can be represented geometrically [23]. Furthermore, Clark and Roche suggest the use of games in fraction learning; the game is done like a monopoly game using a kind of broken board, dice, and involves all students in the class [24].

The use of image representation is suggested by de Castro [25]. The same representation, using colored art drawings was suggested by Scaptura et al. [26]. Fractional learning using technology was suggested by Mendiburo and Hasselbring; they also prove that teaching fractions with technology are as effective as teaching fractions that use physical manipulation [27].

Other researchers, Lesh, Posh, and Behr stated that students gain a better understanding when they can identify and model mathematical concepts through various representations [28]. Furthermore, the Principle and Standards for School Mathematics suggest that students represent their mathematical ideas so that mathematical ideas make sense according to students [29]. One learning model that offers the use of diverse representations is the Lesh Translation Model.

3. Lesh translation model

Lesh Translational Model states that basic mathematical ideas can be represented in 5 ways: real (manipulative) objects, images, real-world contexts, verbal symbols, and written symbols. This model is illustrated by the following **Figure 1**:

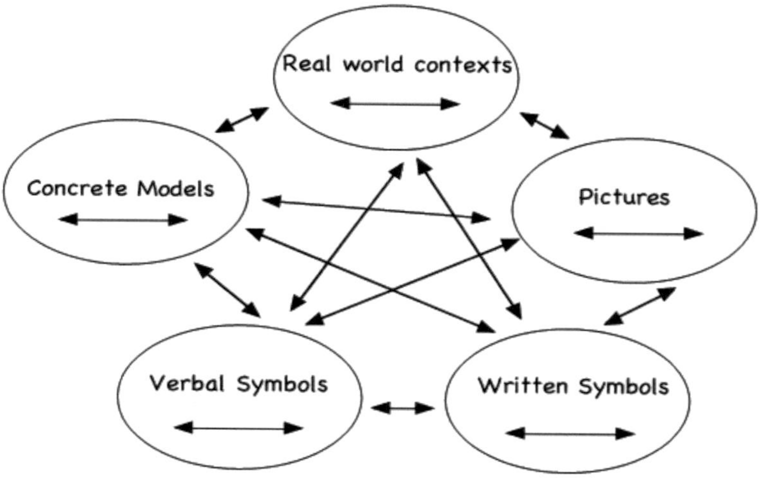

Figure 1.
Lesh translation model [30].

Lesh Translational Model emphasizes interactions within and between representations. The arrows between one representation and another represent the intermodal translation, while the arrows in one mode represent the translation in the mode itself. This model suggests that a good understanding of mathematical ideas requires experience from various modes (ways) and the experience of making connections between and within these modes of representation. A translation requires interpretation of ideas that differ from one mode to another. This activity with its intellectual relations activity reflects dynamic learning.

4. Mental act, ways of thinking, and ways of understanding

According to Harel [31], human reasoning involves many mental actions such as interpreting, guessing, concluding, proving, explaining, compiling, generalizing, applying, predicting, classifying, searching and solving problems. He states that way of understanding is a certain cognitive product of mental actions carried out by an individual. For example, after seeing the symbol $\frac{3}{4}$, one can interpret (one mental action) to produce meaning for the symbol $\frac{3}{4}$. The resulting interpretation is one's Ways of Understanding of the symbol $\frac{3}{4}$. This way of understanding can be different depending on the context, and if judged by an observer, can be considered right or wrong. For example, in a context one can interpret the symbol $\frac{3}{4}$ as "3 objects out of 4 objects," and another person can interpret as "repeated sums: $\frac{1}{4}+\frac{1}{4}+\frac{1}{4}$." Others might be able to produce sophisticated Ways of Understanding such as equivalent classes ($\frac{3n}{4n}$ where n is a non-zero integer) and naive Ways of Understanding, such as "two numbers with a bar between them."

Ways of Thinking is a cognitive characteristic of the Mental Act. The cognitive characteristics of the Mental Act are inferred from observations of Ways of Understanding (cognitive products of mental actions). For example, a teacher who follows students' mathematical behavior might conclude that students' interpretations of mathematical symbols are inflexible, there are absolutely no quantitative views, or for example, students' interpretations of symbols are flexible and connected with other concepts. Another example, the teacher can conclude that students' proof of mathematical statements is based on empirical evidence, or based on deductive reasoning [31].

5. Mental act, ways of thinking, and ways of understanding of MLD student

Here are the results of the data analysis from three students with MLD; we found mental acts, ways of understanding, and ways of thinking as follows:

5.1 Problem solving

Here is one example of student work that used mental act problem-solving (**Figure 2**).

In **Figure 2**, the student solves a problem: a tailor receives $\frac{2}{3}$ m of white cloth with floral motifs to make a handkerchief. Each handkerchief requires $\frac{1}{6}$ m of fabric. How many handkerchiefs can be made?. To solve this problem, the student wrote: $\frac{2}{3}\!:\!\frac{1}{6} = \frac{2}{3} \times \frac{6}{1} = 4$ handkerchiefs. To answer this word problem, the student performs mental act problem-solving by modeling mathematical word problem into fraction division operation. Then he solves the problem of dividing the fraction using the invert multiple algorithm method [32].

A problem-solving approach is a cognitive characteristic of mental act problem-solving. From the results of the analysis of the answers, it was found that 8 students did the problem-solving approach. In the answers above, it appears that students understand the questions and answer them using a problem-solving approach, in the form of an invert multiple algorithm (IMA) strategy in fraction division operations.

The solution is a cognitive product of mental act problem-solving. From the results of the analysis of answers, obtained student answers are examples of the way of understanding solution.

5.2 Interpreting

The second identifiable mental act of MLD students is interpreting. The example of student work is as follows (**Figure 3**).

In **Figure 3**, the student is asked to describe fractions $\frac{1}{2}$ and $\frac{2}{5}$ in two different ways. Students have been able to interpret $\frac{1}{2}$ with two different interpretation, which is the rectangle and triangle picture. In the rectangle picture which is divided into two parts; one part is shaded and the other part is not shaded. In the triangle picture which is divided into two parts; one part is shaded and the other part is not shaded.

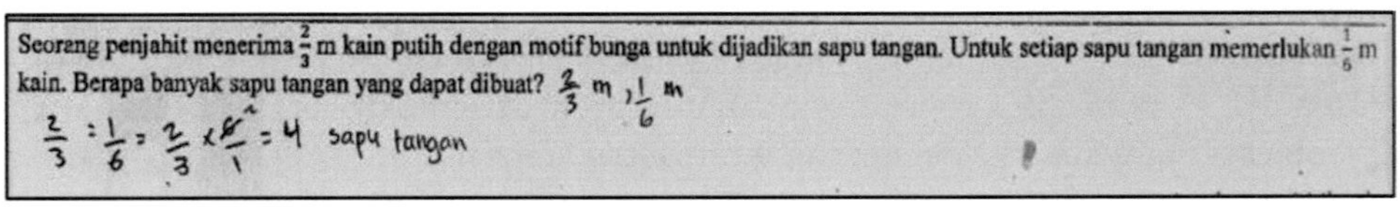

Figure 2.
Mental act problem-solving of MLD student.

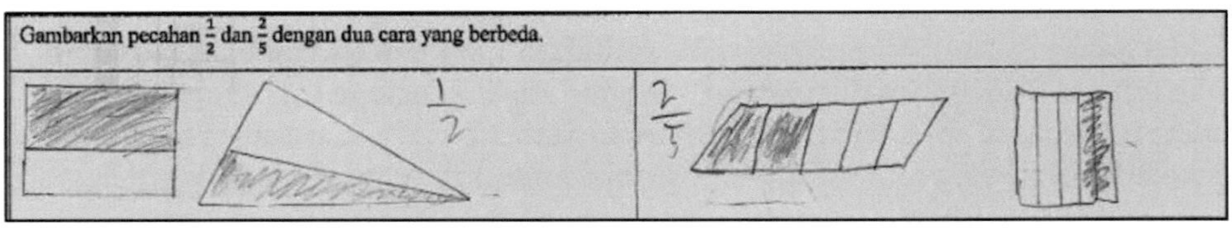

Figure 3.
Mental act interpreting of MLD student.

Mental act	Way of understanding	Way of thinking
Problem-solving	Solution	Problem-solving approach: invert multiply algorithm
Interpreting	Interpretation	Multiple interpretations (as pictures of the square, rectangle, etc.)

Table 1.
The mental act, way of understanding, and way of thinking.

There is something interesting in the triangle picture, students divide the triangle in the centerline, with a horizontal triangle position. Next, students interpret $\frac{2}{5}$ with pictures of parallelograms and squares, each of which is divided into five parts; two parts are shaded and the other is not shaded.

Diverse interpretation of mathematical symbols is a cognitive characteristic of mental act interpreting (way of thinking). From the analysis of MLD student test result data, it was found that he made a fractional interpretation in the form of images, namely rectangular and circular images, as shown above. Interpretation is a cognitive product of mental act interpreting. From the results of the analysis of MLD student answers, it is an embodiment of the way of understanding interpreting, namely interpretation. The students' interpretation of the fractions $\frac{1}{2}$ and $\frac{2}{5}$ is a picture of a rectangle, triangle, parallelogram, and square, as shown above.

We summarize these findings in **Table 1**.

6. The error pattern of MLD students in fractions learning

Some patterns of errors made by MLD students are as follows:

6.1 Students know the common denominator method in the addition of fractions; however, they incorrectly apply the method

The pattern of mistakes of the three students is wrong in applying the denominator equalization procedure. Here is a picture showing this (**Figure 4**).

In the questions, participants are asked to solve two fraction addition questions. In the first problem (part a), students are asked to solve questions $\frac{1}{3}+\frac{1}{3}=....$ This question aims to reveal students' understanding of the fraction addition operation with the same denominator. For this problem, students give the correct answer: $\frac{1}{3}+\frac{1}{3}=\frac{2}{3}$.

In the second problem (part b), students are asked to solve questions $\frac{1}{3}+\frac{1}{2}=....$ This problem aims to reveal students' understanding of the sum of fractions with different denominators. In this problem, students give answers: $\frac{1}{3}+\frac{1}{2}=\frac{1}{6}+\frac{1}{6}=\frac{2}{6}$. Learners already know the procedure to do the denominator in the addition operation of

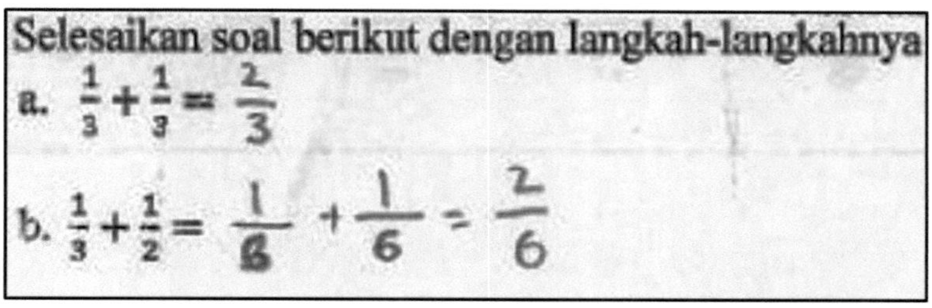

Figure 4.
Example of an error pattern in applying the denominator equalization procedure to the fraction addition operation.

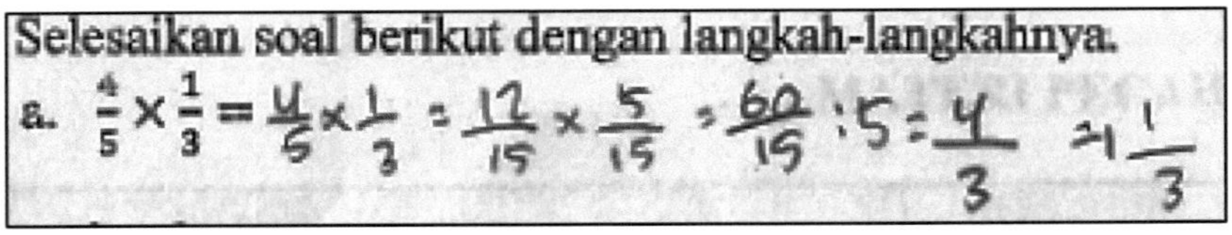

Figure 5.
Example of error pattern applying the denominator equalization procedure to multiplication operations.

fractions. So when he sees the question $\frac{1}{3} + \frac{1}{2} = ...$, he performs the denominator equalization procedure by changing 3 to 6 in the first term and changing 2 to 6 in the second term. However, students do not make numerator changes. So, participants already know the denominator equalization procedure, but do not make adjustments to the numerator. In other words, students mistakenly understand the denominator equalization procedure in fraction addition operations.

6.2 Students use the common denominator approach (for fraction addition) in the multiplication of fraction

The second error pattern is very interesting, namely, students apply the denominator equalization procedure in multiplication operations. Here is a picture showing this (**Figure 5**).

In the problem, students are asked to solve questions $\frac{4}{5} \times \frac{1}{3} = ...$This problem aims to reveal students' understanding of fraction multiplication. In this problem, students give answers: $\frac{4}{5} \times \frac{1}{3} = \frac{12}{15} \times \frac{5}{15} = \frac{60}{15} \div 5 = \frac{4}{3} = 1\frac{1}{3}$. There is an interesting thing, students apply the denominator equalization procedure (supposed to be the sum operation) on the fraction multiplication operation. So when he saw the problem $\frac{4}{5} \times \frac{1}{3} = ...$, he did the procedure of equating the denominator in the first syllable by changing 5 to 15 and in the second syllable changing 3 to 15. There were other interesting things done by students. He only did the multiplication, namely: $\frac{12}{15} \times \frac{5}{15} = \frac{60}{15}$. He then divides $\frac{60}{15}$ by 5 to produce $\frac{4}{3}$ fractions. The interesting thing is that students apply the denominator equalization procedure in fraction multiplication operations.

6.3 In the division of fraction, students mistakenly apply the invert multiply algorithm

The third error pattern is very interesting, namely, students turn the first syllable in a fraction division operation. Here is a picture showing this (**Figure 6**):

In the second problem (part b), students are asked to solve questions $\frac{9}{4} \div \frac{3}{5} = ...$ This question aims to reveal students' understanding of fraction distribution operations. In this problem, students seem to already know the procedure of division

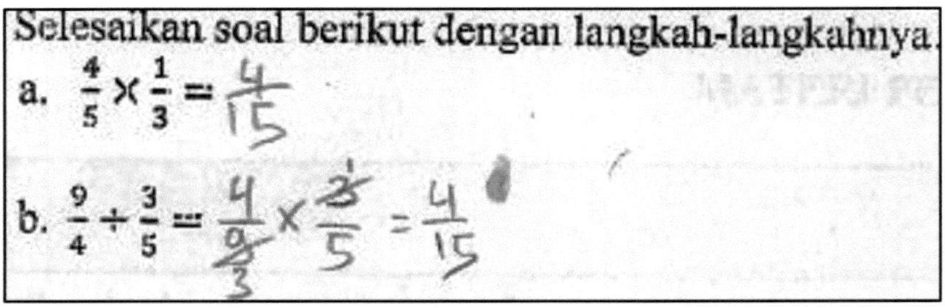

Figure 6.
Example of the first syllable error pattern in a fraction division operation.

operations on fractions. But there is an interesting thing, students use the method of multiplying with the inverse (invert multiply algorithm), but what is reversed is not the second term, but the first term. Consider the following illustration of student answers: $\frac{9}{4} \div \frac{3}{5} = \frac{4}{9} \times \frac{3}{5} = \frac{4}{15}$. So that the answers obtained are reversed, the answer should be $\frac{15}{4}$, students get $\frac{4}{15}$.

7. Discussion

MLD students solve fractions problem procedurally, they apply common denominator approach, drawing a picture, direct multiplied strategy, and invert multiply algorithm in solving fractions problems. They cannot practice the other strategies like using a benchmark or residual which demands the ability to infer and explain. Therefore, we conclude MLD students only perform two mental acts, which are problem-solving and interpreting. They could not develop other mental acts like explaining or inferring.

Some interesting findings when MLD students solve fractions problem are: (1) they know the procedure of common denominator approach in fraction addition operation, however, they mistakenly apply the procedure; (2) in multiplication and divisions operation, they are familiar with the procedure, however, they mistakenly apply the procedure. The two finding is in line with Newton et al. research, they revealed that the main pattern of error in fraction understanding on MLD students is the use of traditional false algorithms [14]. These findings also in accordance with the research of Mazzocco et al., which show that the difficulties in fraction learning are still felt by MLD students until they are in grade 8 [16]. Other researchers also had the same research result, which stated that MLD students make a mistake in performing arithmetic calculations [7].

Another previous research explained that students with MLD have a different ways of thinking in understanding fractions. Lewis considered that the MLD students did not mean to have a lack of understanding of fractions; however, they had different ways of thinking in understanding fractions [11]. We find that MLD students have different ways of thinking in understanding fractions addition operation; they differently understand the common denominator approach, they do not multiply the numerator by the same number with the denominator.

The other research findings deduced that adolescent MLD students are experiencing difficulties in fraction comparison subjects, either fractions comparisons with the same denominator or in fractions comparisons involving a half fraction [12]. Lewis suggested to investigating younger MLD students as the subject. We involved younger students with MLD in our research, a similar result is found, that is MLD students have difficulties in solving fractions comparison problems [33].

In our finding, partitioning activities, which are beneficial for regular students, but not necessarily helpful to MLD students; this may happen because MLD students do not follow a developmental pattern like their regular peers. In accordance with our findings, Lewis explained that partitioning activity was probably the root of understanding the quantity of fractions in regular students; MLD students may not follow this pattern of development [10].

According to Brousseau, the appearance of learning obstacle in mathematics can be caused by three obstacles, namely ontogenic obstacle (mental learning readiness), didactical obstacle (obstacle from teacher instruction or teaching material), and epistemological obstacle (students' knowledge which has limited application context) [34]. In the context of Brousseau theory, the three error patterns of the MLD students in fractions learning is prone to the type of epistemological obstacle, that is MLD students already know fractions concept, however, they have limited application context to the other fractions problems [35].

8. Conclusion

We found only two mental acts with corresponding WoU and WoT, namely problem-solving and interpreting. On the analysis of MLD students, it was found an interesting thing in the mental act problem solving, i.e., the student knew the common denominator approach in the operation of fraction addition, but the practice is still wrong. The same thing is also found in multiplication and division operation. Surprisingly, students use the common denominator approach in the fraction multiplication. In the division of fraction, students mistakenly apply the invert multiply algorithm.

The results of this study can be used by the teachers as a guideline when teaching fractions to students. Future research is recommended to analyze the error patterns of MLD students with other topics in mathematics, such as geometry.

Author details

Suprih Widodo[1*] and Trisno Ikhwanudin[2,3]

1 Universitas Pendidikan Indonesia (Indonesia University of Education), Indonesia

2 Postgraduate Program, Universitas Pendidikan Indonesia (Indonesia University of Education), Indonesia

3 PPPPTK TK dan PLB (Special Teacher Development Center), Indonesia

*Address all correspondence to: supri@upi.edu

References

[1] Strauss V. Trying to figure out why math is so hard for some, theories abound: Genetics, gender, how It's taught. The Washington Post. 2003;**2003**

[2] Adler B. What Is Dyscalculia. Cognitive Center in Sweden: Sweden; 2001

[3] National Center for Learning Disabilities. The State of Learning Disabilities. New York: NCLD; 2014

[4] Geary DC. Mathematics and learning disabilities. Journal of Learning Disabilities. 2004;**37**(1):4-15

[5] Piazza M, Facoetti A, Trussardi AN, Berteletti I, Conte S, Lucangeli D, et al. Developmental trajectory of number acuity reveals a severe impairment in developmental dyscalculia. Cognition. 2010;**116**:33-41

[6] Mazzocco MMM, Feigenson L, Halberda J. Impaired acuity of the approximate number system underlies mathematical learning disability (dyscalculia). Child Development. 2011;**82**:1224-1237

[7] Geary DC, Hoard MK, Byrd-Craven J, DeSota MC. Strategy choices in simple and complex addition: Contributions of working memory and counting knowledge for children with mathematical disability. Journal of Experimental Child Psychology. 2004;**88**:121-151

[8] Mazzocco MMM, Devlin KT, McKenney SJ. Is it a fact? Timed arithmetic performance of children with mathematical learning disabilities (MLD) varies as a function of how MLD is defined. Developmental Neuropsychology. 2008;**33**:318-344

[9] Lewis KE, Fisher MB. Taking stock of 40 years of research on mathematical learning disability: Methodological issues and future directions. Journal for Research in Mathematics Education. 2016;**47**(4):338-371

[10] Lewis KE. Beyond error patterns: A sociocultural view of fraction comparison errors in students with mathematical learning disabilities. Learning Disability Quarterly. 2016b;**1**(14):1-14

[11] Lewis KE. Difference not deficit: Reconceptualising mathematics learning disabilities. Journal for Research in Mathematics Education. 2014;**45**(3)

[12] Lewis KE. Understanding mathematical learning disabilities as developmental difference: A fine-grained analysis of one student's partitioning strategies for fractions. Journal of Education and Development. 2016;**39**(4):812-857

[13] Hunt JH et al. Initial understandings of fraction concepts evidenced by students with mathematical learning disabilities and difficulties: A framework. Learning Disability Quarterly. 2016;**13**(1):1-13

[14] Newton et al. An examination of the ways that students with learning disabilities solve fraction computation problems. The Elementary School Journal. 2014;**115**(1):1-21

[15] Shin M, Bryant DP. Improving the fraction word problem solving of students with mathematics learning disabilities: Interactive computer application. Remedial and Special Education. 2016;**38**(2):76-86

[16] Mazzocco M et al. Limited knowledge of fraction representations differentiates middle school students with mathematics learning disability (dyscalculia) versus low mathematics achievement. Journal of Experimental Child Psychology. 2013;**115**(2):371-387

[17] Gersten R, Chard D, Jayanthi M, Baker S, Morphy P, Flojo J. Mathematics Instruction for Students with Learning Disabilities or Difficulty Learning Mathematics: Asynthesis of the Intervention Research. Portsmouth, NH: RMC Research Corporation, Center on Instruction; 2008

[18] Tian J, Siegler RS. Fractions learning in children with mathematics difficulties. Journal of Learning Disabilities. 2016;**50**(6):614-620

[19] Clarke C, Fisher W, Marks R, Ross S, Zbiek RS. Developing Essential Understanding of Rational Numbers for Teaching Mathematics in Grades 3-5. Reston, VA: NCTM; 2010

[20] Hiebert J, Wearne D. Procedures over concepts: The acquisition of decimal number knowledge. In: Hiebert DJ, editor. Conceptual and Procedural Knowledge: The Case of Mathematics. Hillsdale, NJ: Lawrence Erlbaum Associates; 1986. pp. 199-223

[21] Riccomini PJ. Core Issues of Math: Number Sense and Fraction. Kansas MTSS Symposium. 2010. Available from: www.kansasmtss.org/2010Symposium/Riccomini_Number_Sense_and_Fractions

[22] Wyberg T, Whitney SR, Cramer KA, Monson DS, Leavitt S. Unfolding fraction multiplication: Helps students understand an important algorithm by using a piece of paper and a number line. Mathematics Teaching in The Middle School. 2012;**17**(5):289-293

[23] Dey K, Dey R. Teaching arithmetic of fractions using geometry. Journal of Mathematics Education. 2010;**3**(2):170-182

[24] Clarke D, Roche A. The power of a single game to address a range of important ideas in fraction learning. In: The Australasian Mathematical Psychology Conference 2010, Australia. p. 2010

[25] de Castro BV. Cognitive models: The missing link to learning fraction multiplication and division. Asia Pacific Education Review. 2008;**9**(2):101-112

[26] Scaptura C, Suh J, Mahaffey G. Masterpieces to mathematics: Using art to teaching fraction, decimal, and percent equivalents. Mathematics Teaching in The Middle School. 2007;**13**(1):24-28

[27] Mendiburo M., Hasselbring T. Technology's Impact on Fraction Learning: An Experimental Comparison of Virtual and Physical Manipulative. SREE Conference Abstract Template; 2011

[28] Lesh R, Post T, Behr M. Representations and translations among representations in mathematics learning and problem solving. Problem of representation in the teaching and learning of mathematics. In: Javier C, editor. Hillsdale. NJ: Lawrence Erlbaum Associates; 1987. pp. 33-40

[29] National Council of Teachers of Mathematics. Principles and Standards for School Mathematics. Reston, VA: NCTM; 2000

[30] Cramer K. Using a translation model for curriculum development and classroom instruction. In: Lesh R, Doerr H, editors. Beyond Constructivism: Models and Modeling Perspectives on Mathematics Problem Solving, Learning, and Teaching. Mahwah, NJ: Lawrence Erlbaum Associates; 2003. pp. 449-464

[31] Harel G. What is mathematics? A pedagogical answer to a philosophical question. In: Gold B, Simons RA, editors. Proof and Other Dilemmas: Mathematics and Philosophy. Washington, DC: MAA; 2008. pp. 265-290

[32] Zembat IO. An alternative route to teaching fraction division: Abstraction of common denominator

algorithm. International Electronic Journal of Elementary Education. 2015;**7**(3):399-422

[33] Ikhwanudin T, Suryadi D. How students with mathematics learning disabilities understands fraction: A case from the Indonesian inclusive school. International Journal of Instruction. 2018;**11**(3):309-326. DOI: 10.12973/iji.2018.11322a

[34] Brousseau G. Theory of Didactical Situations in Mathematics. Dordrecht: Kluwer Academic Publishers; 2002

[35] Ikhwanudin T, Prabawanto S, Wahyudin. The error pattern of students with mathematics learning disabilities in the inclusive school on fractions learning. International Journal of Learning, Teaching and Educational Research. 2019;**18**(3):75-95. DOI: 10.26803/ijlter.18.3.5

Section 3

Learning Disabilities Comorbid with Behavioral, Developmental Disorders and Autism

Chapter 7

ADHD as a Specific Cause for Learning Disability

Nada Pop-Jordanova

Abstract

In the spectrum of possible causes for discrepancy between the capacity to learn and the level of school achievement, Attention Deficit Hyperactivity Disorder (ADHD) has an important place. The aim of this chapter is to present obtained own results for a group of 200 pupils, mean age 10.5 ± 2.35 years, and both genders, diagnosed as ADHD following DSM-5 criteria. As psychometric tests, Kohs Block Design Test, Achenbach CBCL, ACTeRS, Stroop Color Word Task (SCWT), and Wisconsin Card Sorting Test (WCST) are used. Additionally, Q-EEG recording using Mitsar 19-channel Q-EEG 201 system was performed. Obtained results confirmed the diagnosis of ADHD as well as the presence of serious difficulties in executive system functioning through ERP's component extracted from Q-EEG analysis. In the chapter, results for Q-EEG will be discussed more extensively including subtypes. As a used nonpharmacological therapeutic approach, very positive outcome of neurofeedback treatment of these children is accentuated.

Keywords: learning problems, ADHD, psychometric tests, Q-EEG, neurofeedback

1. Introduction

Being nonattentive, nonpatient, and enable to follow the teacher instructions during classes, children with Attention Deficit Hyperactivity Disorder (ADHD) represent a huge problem in the educational process. They have additionally variety of learning difficulties.

ADHD is a clinically heterogeneous neurobehavioral disorder associated with tremendous financial costs, stress to families, adverse academic, and occupational outcomes. In adult period, this condition is not totally overcome and stay as a huge risk for addiction, dangerous behavior, unsuccessful occupation, high rate of divorces, etc.

The diagnostics of this condition change in different periods of time. As "a minimal brain damage" or as "minimal brain dysfunction," the condition was named till the 1994, where for the first time, it was renamed as Hyperkinetic Disorder. Three main symptoms, inattention, impulsivity, and hyperactivity, are listed in both manuals, the International Classification of Diseases (ICD-10) where the disorder is named as "Hyperkinetic Disorder" (HKD) and the fourth edition of the Diagnostic and Statistical Manual of Mental Disorders (DSM-IV) where it is named as Attention Deficit Hyperactivity Disorder (ADHD). In DSM-IV, the diagnostic includes three different groups of children: the predominantly Hyperactive-Impulsive Type, the predominantly Inattentive Type, and the Combined Type of ADHD. It was approved that this disorder is more frequently found in boys [1] with the ratio of boys to girls being approximately 4:1 for all three subgroups [2].

In May 2012, American Psychological Association was revising the Fourth Edition of the Diagnostic and Statistical Manual of Mental Disorders, which included some changes in the section on specific learning disabilities. Consequently, DSM-5 considers Specific Learning Disability (SLD) as a type of Neurodevelopmental Disorder that delays the ability to learn or use specific academic skills (e.g., reading, writing, or arithmetic). In this context, SLD is a clinical diagnosis that is not necessarily synonymous with "learning disabilities" used mainly within the education system. SLD characterizes the specific manifestations of learning difficulties at the time of assessment in three major academic domains, namely reading, writing, and mathematics. The group of entities named as "Other Neurodevelopmental Disorders" includes Intellectual Disability, Autism Spectrum Disorder, Attention-Deficit/Hyperactivity Disorder, and Communication Disorders and Motor Disorders. Consequently, whatever criteria for diagnostics are followed, ADHD stays as a huge cause for learning problems.

The differences in diagnostic criteria following different manuals have influenced to the different prevalence rates. As a result, HKD is estimated to be present in approximately 0.5% of children, whereas ADHD has been reported in between 5 and 11.4% of the population [3]. The differences in diagnostics have important implications for both, diagnosis and treatment, because depending on which criteria are used, a child may or may not be considered to have a clinical disorder, which subsequently will influence on the decision about his/her involvement in the school process as well as the need of some treatment.

Many researchers mentioned that ADHD in reality represents a continuum from normal to abnormal behavior. Especially, behavioral studies of children with a predominance of inattentive type have found these children to have some specific problems. For example, inattentive children are less impulsive and less manifest conduct problems than hyperactive children. By contrast, they are more anxious, socially withdrawn, and shy and have more internalizing symptoms. Additionally, they present more frequently academic underachievement and learning problems. Inattentive children are easily confused, stare frequently, often daydream, and they are lethargic, hypoactive, and passive, which are not common in hyperactive children. More specifically, in inattentive children, it was approved deficits in speed of information processing and in focused or selective attention, whereas in the combined type of ADHD, the problem of sustained attention (persistence) and distractibility is more characteristic. These findings suggested that maybe inattentive children should be treated as special group of disorder and not be considered only as a form of ADHD [4].

Although genetic markers in the identification of children with ADHD were not jet found, it was proven that dopamine-related genes are involved in the pathogenesis (such as D1, D2, and D4) [5, 6]. Some form of heredity is additionally confirmed with the fact that this condition could be present in the same family members, especially in twins [7]. In a few recent findings, it was showed that attention deficit hyperactivity disorder (ADHD) shares similar genetic roots and brain structure with autism and obsessive-compulsive disorder (OCD). The impulsivity is characteristic behavior in all three conditions. Additionally, the brain architecture in these conditions presents abnormal findings especially in the structure of the corpus callosum, together with widespread disruptions in white matter. However, children with OCD present fewer structural alterations in comparison with those with autism or ADHD. It is the possible reason that children with autism as well as ADHD manifest earlier specific symptoms in comparison with OCD, which could have a start even in adolescence. Some rare genetic variants associated with autism and schizophrenia also increase a person's chance of having attention deficit hyperactivity disorder (ADHD) [8, 9].

Performing genetic analysis, eight copy number variants (CNVs) are identified, which are more common in people with ADHD than in those without this problem. These same CNVs are also implicated in autism and schizophrenia. In this context, the new hypothesis arises that autism, schizophrenia, and ADHD could have similar biological underpinnings [10]. However, findings do not approve susceptibility genes of larger effect for ADHD, but they can identify genes of smaller effect. Whole genome linkage studies have provided some interesting results for chromosomal regions that need to be further investigated.

The complexity of the ADHD phenotype combined with some genetic findings suggests that identifying endophenotype may be a useful strategy for exact diagnosis. An endophenotype, i.e., intermediate phenotype, is defined as a quantitative biological trait, which is heritable, is reliable in reflecting the function of a discrete biological system, and is presumed to be more closely related to the genetic cause of the disease than the clinical phenotype. The integration of these two approaches (endophenotype and genetic variants) will possibly yield to more definitive results. In this context, increased theta power in EEG record is supposed to be a candidate biological marker of genetic risk for ADHD [11].

In order to find possible neurologic basis for ADHD, many imaging techniques are used. Positron Emission Tomography confirmed that brain metabolism in children with ADHD is lower in the areas responsible for the attention, social judgment, and movement. It is confirmed also with fMRI, SPECT, or BOLD techniques. However, Q-EEG recording appeared to be more available, inexpensive, and useful indicator of brain metabolic activity. It is confirmed that low metabolic activity in the area that generates the corresponding EEG signals is characterized by increasing the slow activities (delta and theta waves) and decreasing the fast beta activities. Strong evidence for the usefulness of the Q-EEG in the diagnostic assessment of ADHD comes from a study performed by Monastra and his team [12, 13].

Many studies confirmed that the main brain system, which is impaired in ADHD, is the executive system. Two parameters are specific for the executive system: (1) arousal, as a generalized activation of the system and (2) attention/focused activation of the system, associated with working memory, action selection, action inhibition, and action monitoring.

As was mentioned before, endophenotype is becoming an important concept in the study of ADHD. The endophenotype in psychiatry can be categorized as anatomical, developmental, electrophysiological, metabolic, sensory, or psychological/cognitive. In this way, endophenotype represents simpler indicator for genetic mechanism than the visible behavioral symptoms. It helps to define subtypes of a particular disorder and can be used as a quantitative trait in genetic analysis of proband and families. In this way, Q-EEG spectrum classification of ADHD population has been developed, defining four main endophenotypes: I subtype where abnormal increase of delta-theta frequency range centrally or centrally frontally is dominant; II subtype where abnormal increase of frontal midline theta rhythm is present; III subtype with an abnormal increase of beta activity frontally; and IV subtype characterized with an excess of alpha activities at posterior, central, or frontal lobes [14].

Still, the complexity of ADHD influences on the underdiagnoses or misdiagnosis of this condition in many school children. Contrary, some hyper diagnostics are also possible. For example, in my research, many gifted children obtained the diagnosis as ADHD because the usual school program for them has been boring, and they manifested hyperactive behavior. The misdiagnose could be also the result of many comorbid disorders, which accompanied ADHD such as conduct problems, high general anxiety, depression, speech problems, autism spectrum disorder, or epilepsy. In this situation, the true ADHD could be overlapped by other similar conditions. From a neuropsychological perspective, comorbidity is considered to be the result of the same brain and cognitive mechanisms involved in attentional and behavioral regulations.

2. Sample and methods

The aim of this chapter is to present own results for a group of 200 pupils, mean age 10.5 ± 2.35 years, and both genders, diagnosed as ADHD. The majority of examinees are boys (85%) manifesting deficit of attention and concentration together with hyperactivity. In girls, the inattention was the main problem. In all of them, school achievement was less than it was been expected by parents and teachers.

Beside interview and clinical examination, the diagnosis is made by multidisciplinary team (pediatrician, neurologist, and psychologist), according criteria noted in DSM-5 manual. All children were tested with Kohs Block Design Test, the Stroop Color Word Task (SCWT), and Wisconsin Card Sorting Test (WCST) and recorded with Q-EEG. Mothers fulfilled Child Behavior Checklist (CBCL) and ADD-H: Comprehensive Parent Rating Scale (ACTeRS). Obtained results are compared with the results for control group, which is consisted of 50 healthy children matched by age and gender.

The Child Behavior Checklist (CBCL) [15], fulfilled by mothers, contains 113 questions related to depression, social communication or withdrawal, somatic complaints, some schizoid traits, hyperactivity, problems in the psychosexual development, problems in the conduct, problems with the judgment, and level of anxiety. Several forms of this instrument are available depending on the age and gender of the examinees. Symptoms are grouped as internalized and externalized. They reflect a distinction between fearful, inhibited, over controlled behavior and aggressive, antisocial, under controlled behavior. The profile can contribute to a formal diagnosis by showing the degree of child's deviance in behaviors that parents could observe better than clinicians, as well as to help to organize effective therapeutic approach.

ACTeRS [16] is composed of 24 items that measure four separate entities: attention, hyperactivity, social skills, and oppositional behavior. This instrument was developed by researchers at the University of Illinois Institute for Child Behavior and Development. In our research, ACTeRS is fulfilled also by mothers. The instrument shows the level of attention, hyperactivity, social skills, and oppositional behavior presented on percentile scale.

The Kohs Block Design Test [17] is performance test standardized to measure intelligence level for mental ages 3–19. The test is easy and understandable without the need of many verbal explanations. In this context, it is especially valuable for testing those with language and hearing difficulties. The test consists of 16 colored cubes and 17 cards with colored designs, which the subject is invited to replicate. Kohs cubes are used to assess the analytic, synthetic, and logic thinking. Block design test possesses a high degree of correlation and reliability with Binet-Simon IQ test and WISC.

The Stroop Color and Word Test (SCWT) [18] was designed to discover possible organic cause of disorder. It assesses cognitive function and provides diagnostic information on possible brain dysfunction due to organic lesions. The test is quick and easy for administration, and it is based on the facts that reading words are faster than the identification of the presented color. The validity and reliability make it a highly useful instrument.

The Wisconsin Card Sorting Test (WCST) [19] is a neuropsychological test for evaluating the mental flexibility ("set shifting") when the stimulus is changed, e.g., the attention, the working memory, and visual processing.

WCST and SCWT were performed using software named Computer Assisted Neuropsychological Diagnostics and Therapy (CANDIT) developed by the Institute of Neuropsychology, Zurich, Switzerland. Each evaluation of the child takes about 2-h duration.

The electrophysiological assessment was performed with system Mitsar 19-channel QEEG 201 (Mitsar Ltd). Quantitative EEG (Q-EEG) is a collection of quantitative methods designed to process EEG signals. The Q-EEG includes spectral and wavelet analyses of the EEG signals. The recording is made up of two conditions, eyes closed and eyes open, lasting 5 min each. In the following, data were recorded, while subjects were performing a visual continuous performance task (VCPT) from Psytask program designed by the Human Brain Institute in Saint Petersburg, Russia. This program comprises the Go/No Go task, which performance is associated with a group of psychological operations named as executive, such as detection and recognition of the stimulus, refreshing the working memory, initiation, and/or inhibition of the behavior and monitoring of the action results. The duration of the tasks was approximately 22 min. Separate channels for recording a signal from the button were used for monitoring the accuracy of the test performance and measuring the response trial.

Electrodes were placed according to the International 10–20 system using an electrode cap with tin electrodes (Electrocap International Inc.). The input signals referenced to the linked ears were filtered between 0.5 and 50 Hz and digitized at a sampling rate of 250 Hz. The impedance was kept below 5 kΩ for all electrodes. The quantitative data were obtained using WinEEG software.

The results obtained from the psychometric measuring are presented in a form of scores and compared with test norms, adopted by the age and gender of the examinees, and presented in figures and tables. The results are considered to be statistically significant at a significance level of 0.05. The data from the electrophysiological assessment were transformed with Fourier analysis and compared with a normative database, grouped by their age. For calculations in this research, the statistical program STATISTICA 10.0 was used.

3. Results and discussion

(At the beginning of this part, I must confirm that presented results are a compilation of different groups of examinees evaluated at different times, and some of them are published in Macedonian journals).

As a start in the evaluation of children with learning problems, testing the intelligence level is of primary importance. Obtained results are very useful for further evaluation especially for exclusion of the intelligence as a factor for presented problems. Evaluation with Kohs Block Design Test showed that ADHD children have intellectual capacities in the norm (IQ = 96 ± 13.15). Mean school notes were as follows: mathematics 3; language 4.5; and nature and society 3 (range 1–5).

Profile obtained for ACTeRS, fulfilled by mothers, confirmed abnormal scores in the scales for attention, social adaptation, and oppositional behavior (between 10 and 23 percentiles), which corresponds with the core symptoms of the disorder. Boys and girls presented similar results, although boys are more hyperactive than girls (**Figure 1**).

CBCL fulfilled also by mothers showed for boy's accentuated anxiety, depression, social withdrawals, and aggressive behavior. Girls are also with social withdrawals, hyperactive, and manifest delinquent behavior (**Figure 2**).

The Q-EEG assessment generally showed dominant theta activity (4–8 Hz) and deficit of beta activity (16–20 Hz) (**Figure 3**).

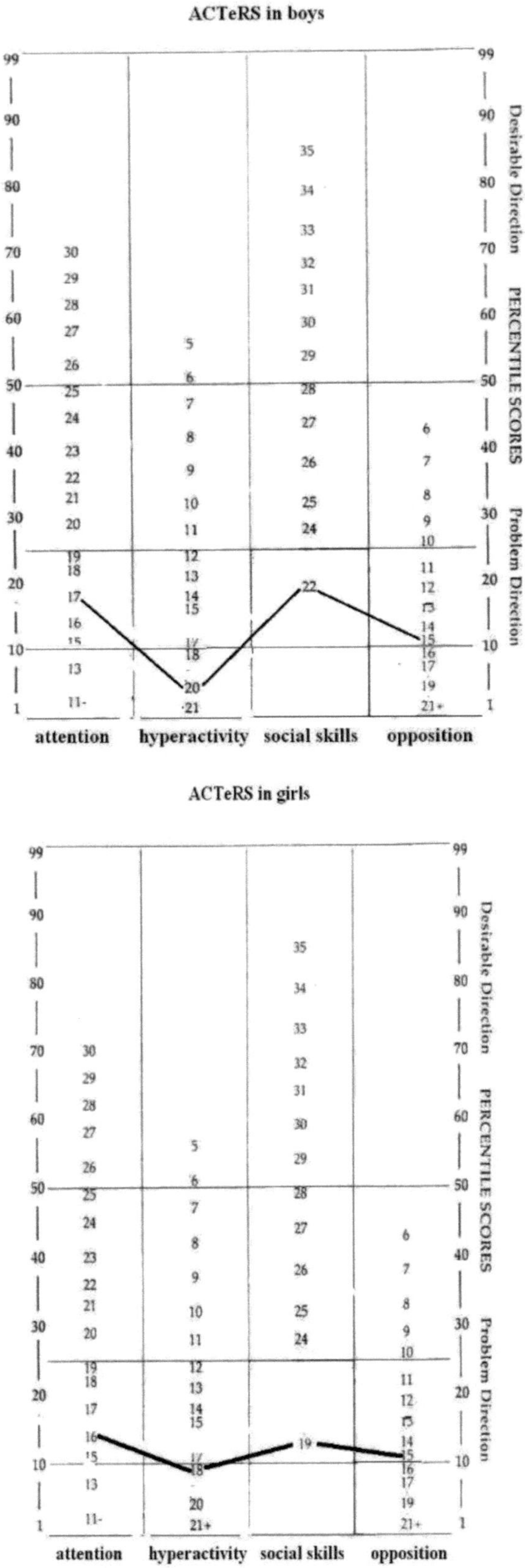

Figure 1.
Profiles obtained for ACTeRS.

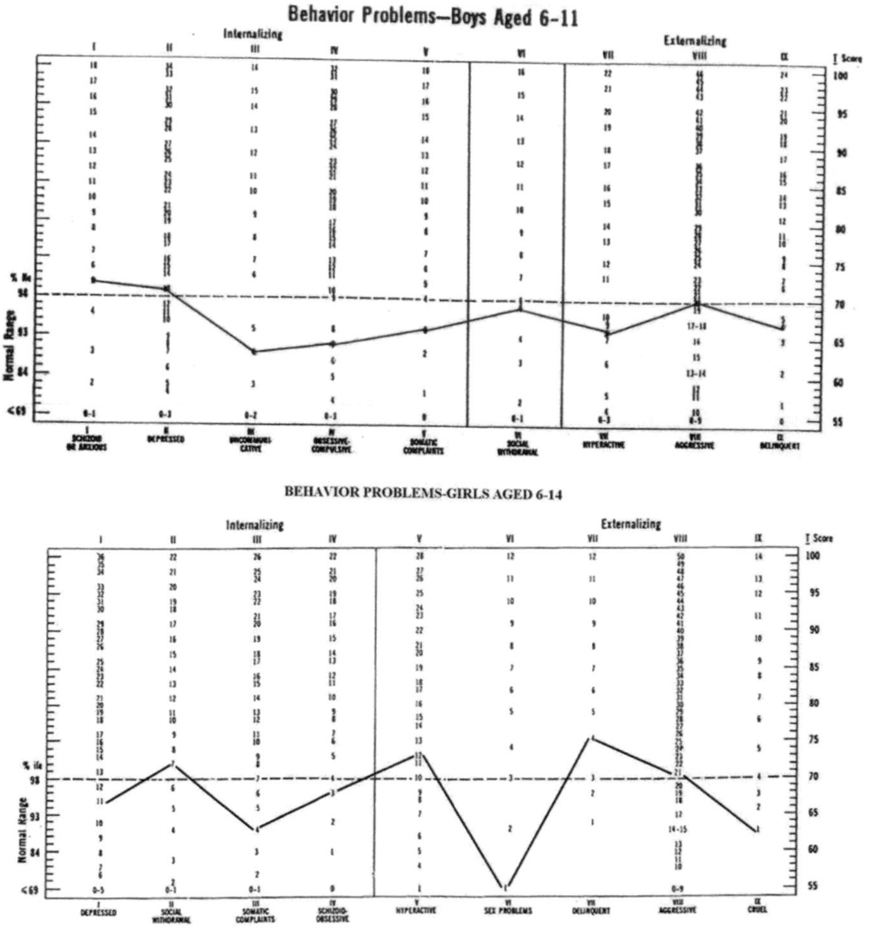

Figure 2.
CBCL profiles for boys and girls.

Theta/beta ratio is presented in **Figure 4**.

The endophenotype presented in Q-EEG records is evaluated according to Kropotov's typology [20]. In Macedonian ADHD children (N = 200), majority (48%) belongs to the combined 1 and 2 subtypes. The other 25% of children showed very slow alpha excess (subtype 4), which corresponds to inattentive form of ADHD mainly found in girls. In another 25%, we found high theta/beta ratio in frontal-central cortex (subtype 1). The subtype 3 with overactive cortex is rarely found in our sample (under 2%).

VCPT, as a part of Q-EEG analysis, showed that hyperactive children performed significantly much omission and commission errors, longer reaction time (RT), and high variation of the reaction time (var RT) compared with test norms (**Table 1**).

The analysis of P3Go component (activation processes) did not showed significant differences concerning the latency and amplitude, while for P3NoGo component (inhibition processes), the latency is not disturbed, but the amplitude is statistically lower (**Table 2**).

Generally, psychometric and psychophysiological evaluation of the examinees confirmed the hyperactivity, average intellectual capacities, and significant number of perseverative and nonperseverative mistakes. Results for VCPT showed significantly higher number of omission and commission errors related to the inattention, shorter reaction time (RT), and higher variation in reaction time (var RT) than test

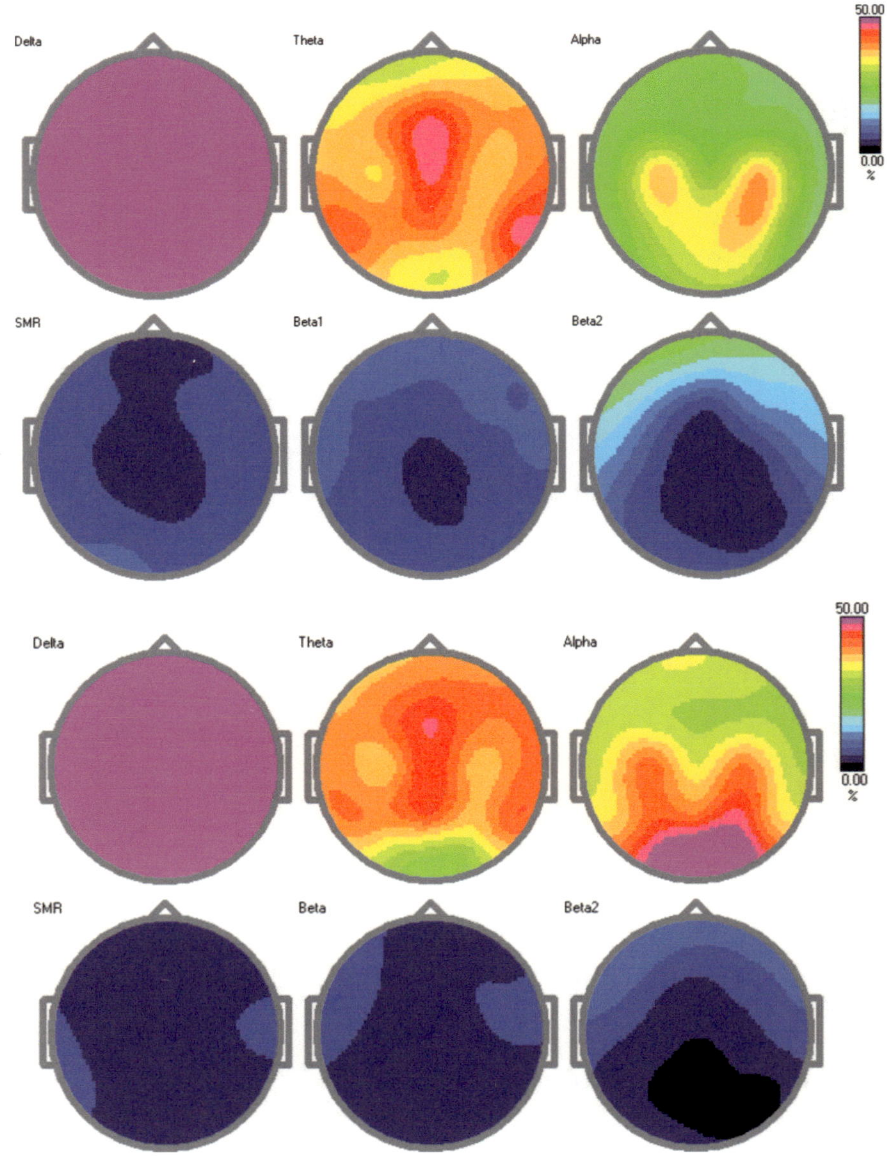

Figure 3.
Average maps of relation of EEG power spectra in ADHD children (EO upper, EC below).

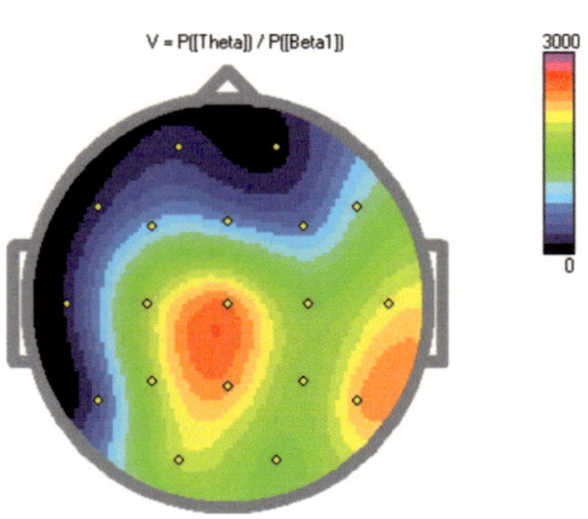

Figure 4.
Theta/beta ratio.

VCPT	ADHD	Norm	t test	p value
Omission errors (Go)	32.25	4	15.65	0.00001*
Commission errors (NoGo)	4.75	1	7.58	0.00000*
RT(ms) Go	456.89	486	−9.17	0.0001*
var RT	18.97	11.7	8.78	0.0000*

$^{*}p < 0.01$.

Table 1.
Results for VCPT in ADHD children.

ERP	ADHD	Norm	t test	p value
P3Go (ms)	327.15	327.89	−0.12	0.9
P3Go (mV)	9.73	8.55	0.77	0.44
P3NoGo (ms)	402.05	415.78	−0.69	0.49
P3NoGo (mV)	4.67	6.23	−2.89	0.006*

$^{*}p < 0.01$.

Table 2.
Components P3Go and P3NoGo in ADHD group.

norms. Values of P3Go component in latency and amplitude are different from the norm, while P3NoGo component showed significant difference in the amplitude.

For better understanding obtained results of analysis, a schematic presentation of components included in executive functions of the brain is shown in **Figure 5**. The components are associated with distinct psychological operations, such as engagement operations (P3bP component), comparison (vcomTL and vcomTR), motor inhibition (P3supF), and monitoring (P4monCC) operations. The ERP results in our evaluated children showed significantly lower amplitude and longer latency for the engagement (P3bP), motor inhibition (P3supF), and monitoring (P4monCC) components, which confirm the executive dysfunction.

In the treatment of our clients, we applied behavior therapy, and especially some biofeedback modalities. Any stimulant medication is not allowed in our country.

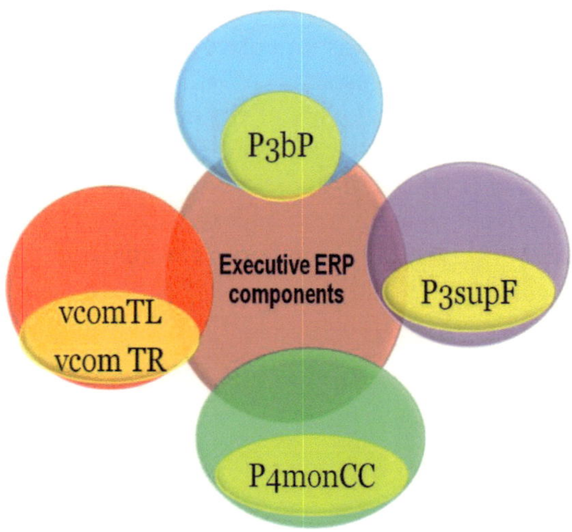

Figure 5.
Executive ERP components.

We introduced biofeedback methodology in 1996 as the first team in our region. Biofeedback is a technique, which helps to learn the control of unaware body's functions (heart rate, dermal activity, muscle tension, peripheral temperature, breathing frequency, brain waves, etc.). Biofeedback could be peripheral or central – neurofeedback. Neurofeedback is a specific behavioral therapy technique used to teach or improve self-regulation of brain activity. The goal of frequency band neurofeedback is to activate a specific brain network.

Common protocol for neurofeedback in many studies comprised diminishing theta activity and optimizing beta brain activity in specific skull points depending on the Q-EEG subtype [21–24]. For our group with ADHD, we used personalized biofeedback protocols depending on the Q-EEG subtype. Generally, we started with 3–5 sessions of electro dermal biofeedback for diminishing anxiety and stress level, and in the following, we used the neurofeedback, two times per week, in the duration of 50 min for each session. **Table 3** shows obtained results before and after biofeedback application in our patients. It is clear that with this kind of therapy, we achieved diminishing of theta, higher power of beta brain waves, changes of theta/beta ratio, and change of brain rate parameter.

In the assessment of ADHD, patient's theta/beta ratio is a parameter used in many studies [24, 25]. The brain rate parameter is indicator introduced by Pop-Jordanova N. and Pop-Jordanov J. for the evaluation of general mental arousal [26, 27]. The values of this parameter are approved in other studies performed in our country [28–30].

The most commonly reported finding in electrophysiological studies of children with ADHD is increased low frequency activity (predominantly theta) compared with age-matched normal controls. Our results are similar and correspond to the previous research examining electrophysiological measures in children and adolescents with ADHD compared with normal controls, which generally reported an increase in theta activity [31, 32] and a decrease in beta activity [33].

Having in mind that ADHD is a complex syndrome, the diagnosis must include large neuropsychological assessment to evaluate mainly the executive system because the symptoms could be different from child to child. In this context, the analysis of ERP's component extracted from Q-EEG records is a modern approach in the diagnosis of ADHD showing the difference in amplitude or latencies. Van der Meere [34] supposed that the smaller amplitude of P3 component is the result of smaller ability for the engagement of the child in the task performance. Additionally, Keage et al. [35] obtained shorter latencies of P3 component in ADHD patients. It must be mentioned that the executive system is changeable through the developmental process, which suggests that ADHD could be the result of slower developmental of some neurological parts of the brain. It is the reason why some children overcome hyperactivity and impulsivity with maturation.

In a multicenter study [24], the theta/beta ratio was found to discriminate ADHD patients and normal controls with high sensitivity and specificity. In this context, Snyder and Hall [36] based on meta-analysis concluded that

Parameter	Before NF (μV)	After NF (μV)	*t* test	Significance
Beta brain waves	4.86 ± 1.6	8.0 ± 1.38	5.23	$p < 0.01$
Theta brain waves	20.95 ± 1.38	15.29 ± 1.38	8.47	$p < 0.01$
Theta/beta	4.7 ± 1.38	2.0 ± 1.6	4.5	$p < 0.01$
Brain rate	7.86 ± 0.56	8.22 ± 0.63	6.6	$p < 0.01$

Table 3.
Main parameters before and after neurofeedback training.

the theta/beta ratio has much higher predictive power than rating scales do, for separating ADHD for healthy children. However, the absolute and relative power of theta is higher in young children than in adolescents and adults [20, 37]. High theta/beta ratios and high theta values in ADHD can be interpreted as a result of a developmental delay.

The electrophysiological characteristics of ADHD obtained with Q-EEG recording and recent machine-learning methods promise easy-to-use approaches that can be complementary to the existing diagnostic tools, especially when sufficiently large samples are used. To separate ADHD group from healthy people, neuroalgorithms are used as model for multidimensional brain networks. For this reason, subtypes of ADHD can be used as biomarkers of disorder.

For our own experience, we can conclude that quantitative EEG is a promising approach in diagnostics of this complex disorder. In other words, for diagnostics, it is not enough to listen parents and teachers, but it is imperative to apply a large psychophysiological evaluation of suspected pupils. Q-EEG results can also be helpful in predicting response to stimulant medication and in selecting protocols for neurofeedback. So, we are facing today a renaissance of EEG. On the one hand, the renaissance is associated with obtaining new knowledge regarding neuronal mechanisms of generation of electric neuronal oscillations in spontaneous EEG as well as regarding functional meaning of different waves in event-related potentials [38, 39].

Based on extensive research during the last decade, we now recognize the existence of Q-EEG subtypes in ADHD patients and understand the need of different neurofeedback protocols to correct these abnormalities. However, some of the protocols at the first year of neurofeedback era were obtained empirically without Q-EEG analysis. Most of the protocols use the conventional EEG in the frequency range higher than 0.1 Hz, while EEG at lower frequencies was used in studies of a German group at the University of Tubingen [39].

We can conclude that a Q-EEG allows to the psychologist looking for the brain functioning in easy and cheap way.

In the therapeutic approach, neurofeedback is confirmed as an excellent tool for training certain brain networks and thus improving the behavior, but the therapist is still an indispensable component in the treatment. The support, the instructions, and the presence of the professional in vicinity to the child are a guaranty for success. In some countries (i.e., Israel), different modalities of biofeedback are used in school settings for stress management as well as for training abilities for better achievement. In this context, our team have good experience with peak performance training in school children and in sport [40, 41].

4. Conclusions

- In the vide spectrum of learning disabilities, ADHD takes a large part.
- The diagnosis must be done with the collaboration of teachers, parents, pediatrician, clinical psychologist, and child neuropsychiatrist.
- Different psychometric tests can be used, but they are not sufficient for diagnostics.
- Evaluation of brain dynamics, especially executive functions are inevitable.
- Endophenotype represents simpler indicator to genetic mechanism than the behavioral symptoms and is very important for treatment plan.

- Neurofeedback confirmed its usefulness and cost-benefit as a nonpharmacological treatment. A brain-rate parameter, introduced by our team, appeared to be more realistic in the assessment and the follow up of the obtained results. In the future, we propose to include brain-rate-based neurofeedback training.

Acknowledgements

Many thanks for my collaborators Silvana Markovska-Simoska, PhD, Macedonian Academy of Sciences and Arts, and Tatjana Zorcec, Clinical Psychologist PhD, University Children Hospital, Skopje. They recorded the Q-EEG and give the interpretations. No funding was obtained for this research.

Conflict of interest

The author declares no conflict of interest.

Author details

Nada Pop-Jordanova
Macedonian Academy of Sciences and Arts, Skopje, Republic of North Macedonia

*Address all correspondence to: npopjordanova@ymail.com

References

[1] Gaubb M, Caryn L, Carlsonph D. Gender differences in ADHD: A meta-analysis and critical review. Journal of the American Academy of Child & Adolescent Psychiatry. 1997;**36**(8):1036-1045. DOI: 10.1097/00004583-199708000-00011

[2] de Quirós GB, Kinsbourne M, Palmer RL, Rufo DT. Attention deficit disorder in children: Three clinical variants. Journal of Developmental and Behavioral Pediatrics. 1994;**15**(5):311-319

[3] Scahill L, Schwab-Stone M. **E**pidemiology of ADHD in school-age children. Child and Adolescent Psychiatric Clinics of North America. 2000;**9**:541-555

[4] Barkley R. The inattentive type of ADHD as a distinct disorder: What remains to be done. Clinical Psychology. 2001;**8**(4):489-493. DOI: 10.1093/clipsy.8.4.489

[5] Jaber M, Robinson SW, Missale C, Caron MG. Dopamine receptors and brain function. Neuropharmacology. 1996;**35**(11):1503-1519. DOI: 10.1016/s0028-3908(96)00100-1

[6] Loo S, Hale S, Hanada G, Macion J, Shrestha A, McGough J, et al. Familial clustering and DRD4 effects on EEG measures in multiplex families with attention-deficit hyperactivity disorder. Journal of the American Academy of Child and Adolescent Psychiatry. 2010;**49**(4):368-377

[7] Mick E, Faraone SV. Genetics of attention deficit hyperactivity disorder. Child and Adolescent Psychiatric Clinics of North America. 2008;**17**(2):261-284. DOI: 10.1016/j.chc.2007.11.011

[8] Kushki A, Anagnostou E, Hammill C, et al. Examining overlap and homogeneity in ASD, ADHD, and OCD: A data-driven, diagnosis-agnostic approach. Translational Psychiatry. 2019;**9**:318. DOI: 10.1038/s41398-019-0631-2

[9] Brem S, Grünblatt E, Drechsler R, Riederer P, Walitza S. The neurobiological link between OCD and ADHD. Attention Deficit and Hyperactivity Disorders. 2014;**6**(3):175-202. DOI: 10.1007/s12402-014-0146-x

[10] Ramos-Quiroga JA, Sánchez-Mora C, Casas M, Garcia-Martínez I, Bosch R, Nogueira M, et al. Corrigendum to 'Genome-wide copy number variation analysis in adult Attention-Deficit and Hyperactivity Disorder'. Journal of Psychiatric Research. 2014;**52**:60-67. DOI: 10.1016/j.jpsychires.2014.01.008

[11] Tye C, Rijsdijk F, McLoughlin G. Genetic overlap between ADHD symptoms and EEG theta power. Brain and Cognition. 2014;**87**:168-172. DOI: 10.1016/j.bandc.2014.03.010. [Epub: 19 April 2014]

[12] Monastra V, Lubar J, Linden M. The development of a quantitative electroencephalographic scanning process for attention deficit-hyperactivity disorder reliability and validity studies. Neuropsychology. 2001;**15**:136-144

[13] Monastra V, Lubar J, Linden M, et al. Assessing attention deficit/hyperactivity disorder via quantitative electroencephalography an initial validation study. Neuropsychology. 1999;**13**:424-433. DOI: 10.1037/0894-4105.13.3.424

[14] Kropotov J. Quantitative EEG, ERP's and neurotherapy. Amsterdam: Elsevier Publ; 2009

[15] Achenbach M, Edelbrock C. Manual for the Child Behavior Check List

and Revised Child Behavior Profile. Burlington: University of Vermont; 1983

[16] Ullmann K, Sleator K, Sprague L. Introduction to the use of ACTeRS. Psychopharmacology Bulletin. 1985;**21**:915-919

[17] Kohs' test. Zavod za produktivnost dela. Ljubljana, Slovenia: 1967

[18] Stroop JR. Studies of interference in serial verbal reactions. Journal of Experimental Psychology. 1935;**18**:64662

[19] Anderson SW, Damasio H, Jones RD, Tranel D. Wisconsin card sorting test performance as a measure of frontal lobe damage. Journal of Clinical and Experimental Neuropsychology. 1991;**13**:909-922

[20] Kropotov J, Ponomarev VA. Decomposing N2 NOGO wave of event-related potentials into independent components. Neuroreport. 2009;**20**:1592-1596. DOI: 10.1097/WNR.0b013e3283309cbd

[21] Pop-Jordanova N. Biofeedback application for somatoform disorders and attention deficit hyperactivity disorder (ADHD) in children. International Journal of Medicine and Medical Sciences. 2009;**1**(2):17-22

[22] Pop-Jordanova N, Markovska S, Zorcec T. Neurofeedback treatment of children with attention deficit hyperactivity disorder. Prilozi. 2005;**2**:35-42

[23] Pop-Jordanova N. Chapter 13: QEEG characteristics and biofeedback modalities in children with ADHD. In: Norvilitis JM, editor. Current Directions in ADHD and Its Treatment. Rijeka, Croatia: InTech; 2012. pp. 249-268

[24] Lubar JF. Discourse on the development of EEG diagnostics and biofeedback for attention-deficit/hyperactivity disorders. Biofeedback and Self-Regulation. 1991;**16**(3):201-225. DOI: 10.1007/bf01000016

[25] Monastra V, Monastra D, George S. The effects of stimulant therapy, EEG biofeedback, and parenting style on the primary symptoms of attention-deficit/hyperactivity disorder. Applied Psychophysiology and Biofeedback. 2002;**27**(4):231-249. DOI: 10.1023/A:1021018700609

[26] Pop-Jordanova N, Pop-Jordanov J. Spectrum-weighted EEG frequency ("brain-rate") as a quantitative indicator of mental arousal. Prilozi. 2005;**26**(2):35-42

[27] Pop-Jordanov J, Pop-Jordanova N. Neurophysical substrates of arousal and attention. Cognitive Processing. 2009;**10**(Suppl. 1):S1-S9

[28] Pop-Jordanova N. Chapter 8: Brain Rate as an Indicator of the Level of Consciousness. In: Cvetkovic D, Cosic I, editors. States of Consciousness: Experimental Insights into Meditation, Waking, Sleep and Dreams. Berlin, Heidelberg: Springer; 2011. pp. 187-201

[29] Markovska-Simoska S, Pop-Jordanova N. Quantitative EEG spectrum-weighted frequency (brain rate) distribution in adults with ADHD. CNS Spectrums. 2011;**16**(5):111-119

[30] Demerdzieva A, Pop-Jordanova N. Brain Rate Parameter in Children with General Anxiety Disorder. Pril (Makedon Akad Nauk Umet Odd Med Nauki). 2019;**40**(1):41-50

[31] Mann C, Lubar J, Zimmerman A, Miller C, Muenchen R. Quantitative analysis of EEG in boys with attention deficit hyperactivity disorder: Controlled study with clinical implications. Pediatric Neurology. 1992;**8**:30-36. DOI: 10.1016/0887-8994(92)90049-5

[32] Matsuura M, Okubo Y, Toru M, et al. A cross-national EEG study of children with emotional and behavioral problems: A WHO collaborative study in the Western Pacific Region. Biological Psychiatry. 1993;**34**(1-2):59-65. DOI: 10.1016/0006-3223(93)90257-E

[33] Callaway E, Halliday R, Herning RI. A comparison of methods for measuring event-related potentials. Electroencephalography and Clinical Neurophysiology. 1983, 1983;**55**(2):227-232. DOI: 10.1016/0013-4694(83)90192-X

[34] Van der Meere J. The Role of Attention, Hyperactivity Disorders of Childhood. Cambridge University Press; 1996. pp. 111-148

[35] Keage H, Clark CR, Hermens D, Gordon E. Distractibility in AD/HD predominantly inattentive and combined subtypes: The P3a ERP component, heart rate and performance. Journal of Integrative Neuroscience. 2006;**5**(1):139-158. DOI: 10.1142/S0219635206001070

[36] Snyder SM, Hall JR. A meta-analysis of quantitative EEG power associated with attention-deficit hyperactivity disorder. Journal of Clinical Neurophysiology. 2006;**23**(5):440-455. DOI: 10.1097/01.wnp.0000221363.12503.78

[37] Näätänen R. Attention and Brain Function. PsycINFO Database Record; 1992

[38] Luck S. An introduction to the event-related potential technique. In: A Bradford Book. 2005

[39] Strehl U, Aggensteiner P, Wachtlin D, Brandeis D, Albrecht B, Arana M, et al. Neurofeedback of slow cortical potentials in children with attention-deficit/hyperactivity disorder: A multicenter randomized trial controlling for unspecific effects. Frontiers in Human Neuroscience. 2017;**11**:135. DOI: 10.3389/fnhum.2017.00135. eCollection 2017

[40] Pop-Jordanova N, Cakalaroska I. Comparison of biofeedback modalities for better achievement in high school students. Macedonian Journal of Medical Science. 2008;**1**(2):25-30

[41] Pop-Jordanova N, Demerdzieva A. Biofeedback training for peak performance in sport - Case report. Macedonian Journal of Medical Sciences. 2010;**3**(2):113-118

Chapter 8

Developmental Dyscalculia: Nosological Status and Cognitive Underpinnings

Ricardo Moura, Suzane Garcia and Júlia Beatriz Lopes-Silva

Abstract

Mathematics is one of the main challenges faced by students throughout school life, with long-lasting impact on social life, including employability and incomes. The development of the research on numerical cognition occurred together with the study of math learning and its related deficits, in special developmental dyscalculia (DD). The present chapter explores the literature on DD in two levels. First, we discuss about the nosological status of the disorder together with considerations about its diagnosis. Afterward we review the main research findings regarding the cognitive underpinnings of DD, from numerical representations to domain general processes, including working memory and language.

Keywords: dyscalculia, learning disabilities, dyscalculia diagnosis, numerical cognition, learning

1. Introduction

Living in today's society requires well-developed mathematical competencies. As more cliché as this statement may sound, there is a robust scientific literature indicating that higher mathematical competencies are associated with higher employability and incomes [1–3], profitable financial decisions [4], and even better health outcomes [5]. Despite this well-established body of evidence, many adults and children, even from developed countries, struggle to perform simple arithmetic [6].

The reasons for failing at math are diverse and include socioeconomic [7, 8], educational [9], and emotional factors [10, 11]. Math is a complex and abstract discipline and depends mostly of formal instruction at school. Moreover, mathematical knowledge is also largely cumulative, so that newer, more complex, and abstract concepts depend on previous knowledge, which can either be acquired intuitively, like reciting the sequence of number words, or also formally at school. Therefore, we can say that a great part of the difficulties faced by children when learning or performing math activities are due to the complexity of mathematics itself. It is known that, compared to other disciplines, difficulty in learning math is already observed in children in the first years of school [12].

Some children, nevertheless, show persistent and important difficulties in learning math, which cannot be explained by socioeconomic, emotional, educational, psychiatric, or intellectual factors. In these cases the label developmental dyscalculia (DD) is often applied, and difficulties encompass a broad range of mathematical tasks, like reading and writing numbers in different formats, comparing numbers and quantities, and performing the basic arithmetical operations [7, 13–16]. Some authors also indicate deficits in abilities concerning magnitude representation and the comprehension and use of symbolic codes to represent numerical information [17–19]. The estimates for prevalence of DD vary from 3 to 6% of school-aged children [7, 20, 21].

Despite the relative consensus about what are the difficulties that characterize DD, there is still some debate concerning the diagnostic criteria, neuropsychological underpinnings, and rehabilitation strategies. In the following sections, we will discuss in detail each of these three topics.

2. Nosological status

2.1 Diagnosis

Two main questions concern the diagnosis of DD. The first question is about the diagnostic criteria, and in the literature on the epidemiology of learning disabilities, three approaches are commonly reported. The discrepancy criteria are probably the most common in research studies and define math learning disability from the discrepancy between an average of above- average performance on general cognitive capacity (often the IQ) and the low performance on standardized math tests. The absolute threshold criteria is similar to the discrepancy criteria, but the disability is defined solely by the low performance in a standardized math test. The response to intervention criteria establish the diagnosis after investigating how the child responds to a set of psychopedagogical interventions. In this way, the persistency of the difficulty and not the discrepancy between capacity and performance is the main criteria for diagnosis.

The second main question concerns the definition on how low the performance in an achievement test must be in order to diagnose DD. The cutoff scores frequently used are 30th, 25th, 10th, and 5th percentiles. Higher cutoff scores (25th and 30th percentiles) are less conservative and, naturally, more prone to false positives. Lower cutoff score is more conservative when labeling children and less prone to false positive. Some authors argue that the sample of individuals labeled under higher cutoff scores is more heterogeneous, with their difficulties in math being more attributable to social, educational, and motivational factors and therefore are less stable over time [22]. On the other hand, the individuals whose performance falls into the more conservative cutoff scores are a more homogeneous group, and their difficulties are more probably associated to cognitive factors. Mazzocco [15] suggests that the individuals with performance under the fifth percentile must be identified as DD, and those with performance under the 30th percentile must be identified as "mathematics difficulties."

2.2 Comorbidity and cognitive heterogeneity

The investigation of DD nosology also involves studying its comorbidities with other syndromes and how the cognitive profile varies among individuals. It is estimated that only 30% of the DD children are free of comorbidities [23]. The main comorbidities of DD are with developmental dyslexia and ADHD, with comorbidity rates of 40% for the first [24] and between 25 and 42% for the second [23, 25].

According to Rubinsten and Henik [26], different cognitive deficits can be the cause of difficulties in learning math, with comorbidities being mostly due to a combination of deficits. For example, the pure cases (for which the label DD is applied) are due to a deficit in the abstract representation of number, in the cognitive level, and a deficit in the functioning of the intraparietal sulcus, in the neural level. The comorbidity of dyscalculia and ADHD would be explained by the co-occurrence of deficits in the processing of number and in attentional mechanisms. In turn, comorbidity with dyslexia is due to a single deficit in the angular gyrus that would cause a deficit in associating symbols (Arabic numbers, words) to a meaning. The cases of comorbidity would be referred as mathematics learning difficulties (MLD).

3. Cognitive mechanisms

Following the diversity of activities involved in math and the heterogeneity of manifestations observed in mathematics difficulties, the cognitive mechanisms are also diverse and related to basic numerical representations, working memory, visuospatial reasoning, and language. In the following, the literature on each of these mechanisms will be reviewed in more detail.

3.1 Nonsymbolic representations

Humans, like all other animals, are born with only a rudimentary, language-independent, system dedicated to grasping quantities from the environment [27]. Naturally, this system is not able to process numerical symbols, which are, from a phylogenetic perspective, a very recent cultural invention that demands encultura-tion in order to be assimilated by the human brain [28]. This inherited preverbal number knowledge operates in two forms, which are considered independent subsystems: the object-tracking system (OTS) and the approximate number system (ANS; [27]). The OTS represents small numerosities up to four with high accuracy and reaches its developmental plateau early in development. The ANS, in turn, is responsible for the representation of larger numerosities analogically and, therefore, with increasingly imprecision. One largely accepted model suggests that the ANS represents numbers in an approximate and logarithmically compressed fashion, according to the classical psychophysical laws of Weber and Fechner [29].

Since the last decade, the relationship between basic numerical representations and performance on mathematics has been in the spotlight for many research groups. A handful of evidence has indicated a positive relation between ANS accuracy and math performance [30–37]. Moreover, it has also been shown that children with DD are impaired even in simple tasks that tap ANS representations, such as estimating the numerical size of a set of dots and comparing two sets of dots [17, 38, 39].

A very well-established theory is that DD is the result of a deficit in the foun-dational representations of numbers [14, 26]. For some researchers, this deficitary representation of numbers lies in the ANS [17]. Other researchers, in turn, propose that the deficitary numerical system in DD is the numerosity coding, which is responsible for processing precise, but not continuous, numerical quantities, and in which the whole arithmetical thinking is based on. For a detailed discussion about these hypotheses, see Butterworth [14].

3.2 Symbolic representations

Basic numerical representations are not restricted to nonsymbolic representa-tions. Actually, learning symbolic systems for representing numbers is a landmark in the development of mathematical reasoning. As children learn to speak a sequence of numerical words, they are still devoid of any quantitative meaning [40]. Gradually, these number words are associated with nonsymbolic numerical representations [41, 42]. The mapping between a list of words and their respective numerical representations (meanings) will be established gradually as children become able to perform a range of new tasks. For example, they can use these numeric words to label a set of objects (say "six" when looking to six dolls at a glance). These activities only develop completely around the age of five, when children master the principle of cardinality [43].

Schneider and collaborators [44], in a meta-analysis study, found that the association with performance in arithmetic tests is stronger for symbolic comparison tasks than for the nonsymbolic ones. Furthermore, a find consistently reported by studies indicates that children with DD exhibit weaker performance than controls in tasks requiring comparison of symbolic numbers, like Arabic numbers and number words [18, 38, 45–47]. According to a model proposed by Rousselle and Noël [18], DD can also occur due to a deficit in accessing nonsymbolic representations from numerical symbols (access deficit hypothesis).

3.3 Language

Language influences mathematics in different ways. Many mathematical tasks rely on verbal processing, such as learning the multiplication table, writing and reading numbers, and learning the Arabic code. According to Simmons et al. [48], the relationship between phonological awareness (often measured by a rhyme detection or phoneme elision tasks) and math learning is independent of measures of vocabulary and nonverbal reasoning, thus indicating a genuine verbal-numerical relationship.

Language skills also characterize an important landmark in the development of mathematical abilities. A special case is the ability to convert between numerical notations, often measured by tasks of number writing and number reading, and called number transcoding. Number transcoding is especially important early in school life, since it demands the understanding of basic lexical and syntactic components of Arabic and verbal numerals. As suggested by previous studies, understanding the place-value syntax of Arabic numbers and matching it with number words constitutes a significant landmark that young children must reach in order to succeed in mathematical education [49].

Some scientific evidence suggests that children master the numerical codes after 3 or 4 years of schooling. During the first year of elementary school (around 7-year-old), children still struggle to write and read Arabic numerals [50, 51]. Shortly after, in third and fourth grades (8- and 9-year-old children), most of these difficulties with Arabic numerals are already overcome [38]. This issue was further investigated by Moura et al. [52] in a study using more complex number transcoding tasks and investigating children with and without MLD. Results revealed significant number transcoding difficulties in children with MLD. These difficulties were more prominent in Arabic number writing, but the magnitude of this difference decreased with age, indicating that children with MLD tend to reach the performance of their typical achievers peers. Importantly, from the first to fourth school grades, most of the errors observed in children, regardless of their achievement in mathematics, are well explained by the syntactic complexity of numerals, as most errors were observed in numbers with more digits, and more syntactically complex (like 1002, 4015). A detailed analysis of transcoding errors suggested that children with MLD struggle with the syntactic structure of Arabic numerals, mainly with 3- and 4-digit numbers, until the fourth grade, while typical achievers seem to overcome these difficulties around the third grade. Moreover, the acquisition of lexical primitives seems to be well developed in typical achievers by the first year of elementary school, while children with MLD show a small though significant proportion of lexical errors (e.g., writing *twelve* as 20).

Another important evidence for this interaction between numerical and verbal skills is the high comorbidity between DD and dyslexia. Epidemiological studies indicate that approximately 40% of dyslexic children also have deficits in arithmetic [24]. Some studies suggest comorbidity rates up to 70%, which may be overestimated because of diagnostic criteria and constructs evaluated by standardized arithmetic and reading tests [53]. Importantly, the comorbidity between DD and dyslexia is greater than would be expected by chance if the two entities were fully segregated independently. An influential hypothesis states that children with developmental dyslexia struggle with numerical activities that rely on verbal codes, such as number transcoding and learning arithmetic facts [54].

3.4 Working memory and attention

The association between mathematics skills and working memory and attention has been extensively reported in the literature. In fact, a high variety of numerical tasks including number transcoding, complex calculations, and problem solving require working memory resources and planning. According to Rubinsten and Henik [26], a relevant part of children with DD also present comorbid attention deficit hyperactivity disorder (ADHD) [21, 55].

Interestingly, a brain region that is considered crucial for numerical development, the intraparietal sulcus, is also involved in a range of nonnumerical activities, including attentional control and reasoning [56–59]. Recent studies propose that an important cognitive mark of DD is attentional control. Gilmore et al. [60] found that, due to strategies aiming to control for nonnumerical visual parameters, commonly used dot comparison tasks require inhibitory control mechanisms. Surprisingly, this executive function component is more strongly related to mathematics achievement than the numerical components of magnitude comparison tasks. Similarly, Szucs et al. [61] also proposed that children with DD have more difficulties in inhibiting irrelevant nonnumerical information than their typically developing peers.

3.5 Visuospatial abilities

Together with working memory, visuospatial abilities are one of the most critical abilities related to mathematics achievement, being associated mainly with performance in multidigit calculation, mainly in those requiring borrowing and carry-over procedures [62, 63].

Despite the evidence for a role of visuospatial skills in calculation, a pure visuospatial deficit in children with DD is perhaps less clear than the other cognitive skills discussed above, as there is no well-established visuospatial subgroup of DD. The co-occurrence of mathematics and visuospatial deficits were widely discussed in the context of the so-called nonverbal learning disability [64–66].

If, on the one hand, there is no consensus about a visuospatial deficit in DD, on the other hand, many studies found that children with DD present deficits in the visuospatial component of working memory [61, 67–73]. Importantly, the verbal component of working memory is frequently reported as preserved in these cases [61, 74].

4. Conclusion

Even though the study of the cognitive basis of numerical representations and mathematical performance is relatively new, a consistent body of scientific evidence has already been gathered, allowing important advances in the comprehension of the development of mathematical abilities and in the identification and remediation of mathematical difficulties. Nevertheless, this is a broad field of study and there are still several open questions. Currently, longitudinal and replication studies are especially relevant [75].

Author details

Ricardo Moura[1]*, Suzane Garcia[1] and Júlia Beatriz Lopes-Silva[2]

1 University of Brasília (UnB), Brasília, Brazil

2 Federal University of Minas Gerais (UFMG), Belo Horizonte, Brazil

*Address all correspondence to: ricardoojm@gmail.com

References

[1] Parsons S, Bynner J. Does mumeracy matter more? Education. Institute of Education, University of London: National Research and Development Centre for Adult Literacy and Numeracy; 2006

[2] Dowker A. Individual Differences in Arithmetic: Implications for Psychology, Neuroscience and Education. New York, NY: Psychology Press; 2005

[3] Peters E, Tompkins MK, Knoll MAZ, Ardoin SP, Shoots-Reinhard B, Meara AS. Despite high objective numeracy, lower numeric confidence relates to worse financial and medical outcomes. Proceedings of the National Academy of Sciences. 2019;**116**(39):19386-19391. DOI: 10.1073/pnas.1903126116

[4] Lusardi A, Tufano P. Debt literacy, financial experiences, and overindebtedness. Journal of Pension Economics and Finance. 2015;**14**(4):332-368. DOI: 10.1017/S1474747215000232

[5] Låg T, Bauger L, Lindberg M, Friborg O. The role of numeracy and intelligence in health-risk estimation and medical data interpretation. Journal of Behavioral Decision Making. 2014;**27**(2):95-108. DOI: 10.1002/bdm.1788

[6] OECD. OECD Skills Outlook 2019: Thriving in a Digital World. Paris: OECD Publishing; 2019. DOI: 10.1787/df80bc12-en

[7] Gross-Tsur V, Manor O, Shalev RS. Developmental dyscalculia: Prevalence and demographic features. Developmental Medicine and Child Neurology. 1996;**38**:25-33

[8] Jordan NC, Levine SC. Socioeconomic variation, number competence, and mathematics learning difficulties in young children. Developmental Disabilities Research Reviews. 2009;**15**(1):60-68

[9] Hattie J. Visible Learning: A Synthesis of over 800 Meta-Analyses Relating to Achievement. New York: Routledge; 2008

[10] Hembree R. The nature, effects, and relief of mathematics anxiety. Journal for Research in Mathematics Education. 1990;**21**(1):33. DOI: 10.2307/749455

[11] Carey E, Hill F, Devine A, Szücs D. The chicken or the egg? The direction of the relationship between mathematics anxiety and mathematics performance. Frontiers in Psychology. 2016;**6**:1987. DOI: 10.3389/fpsyg.2015.01987

[12] Mazzocco MMM, Hanich LB, Noeder MM. Primary school age students' spontaneous comments about math reveal emerging dispositions linked to later mathematics achievement. Child Development Research. 2012;**170**:310. DOI: 10.1155/2012/170310

[13] Butterworth B. Developmental dyscalculia. In: Campbell JID, editor. Handbook of Mathematical Cognition. New York, NY, US: Psychology Press; 2005. pp. 455-467

[14] Butterworth B. Foundational numerical capacities and the origins of dyscalculia. Trends in Cognitive Sciences. 2010;**14**(12):534-541. DOI: 10.1016/j.tics.2010.09.007

[15] Mazzocco MMM. Defining and differentiating mathematical learning disabilities and difficulties. In: Berch DB, Mazzocco MMM, editors. Why Is Math So Hard for some Children? The Nature and Origins of Mathematical Learning Difficulties and Disabilities. Baltimore: Brookes; 2007. pp. 29-47

[16] American Psychiatric Association. Diagnostic and Statistical Manual of Mental Disorder. 5th ed. Washington, DC: Author; 2013

[17] Piazza M, Facoetti A, Trussardi AN, Berteletti I, Conte S, Lucangeli D, et al. Developmental trajectory of number acuity reveals a severe impairment in developmental dyscalculia. Cognition. 2010;**116**(1):33-41. DOI: 10.1016/j.cognition.2010.03.012

[18] Rousselle L, Noël MP. Basic numerical skills in children with mathematics learning disabilities: A comparison of symbolic vs non-symbolic number magnitude processing. Cognition. 2007;**102**(3):361-395. DOI: 10.1016/j.cognition.2006.01.005

[19] Wilson AJ, Dehaene S. Number sense and developmental dyscalculia. In: Coch D, Dawson G, Fischer KW, editors. Human Behavior, Learning, and the Developing Brain: Atypical Development. New York, NY, US: The Guilford Press; 2007. pp. 212-238

[20] Reigosa-Crespo V, Valdés-Sosa M, Butterworth B, Estévez N, Rodríguez M, Santos E, et al. Basic numerical capacities and prevalence of developmental dyscalculia: The Havana survey. Developmental Psychology. 2012;**48**:123-135. DOI: 10.1037/a0025356

[21] von Aster MG, Shalev RS. Number development and developmental dyscalculia. Developmental Medicine & Child Neurology. 2007;**49**:868-873

[22] Murphy MM, Mazzocco MMM, Hanich LB, Early MC. Cognitive characteristics of children with Mathematics Learning Disability (MLD) vary as a function of the cutoff criterion used to define MLD. Journal of Learning Disabilities. 2007;**40**(5):458-478. DOI: 10.1177/00222194070400050901

[23] Desoete A. Co-morbidity in mathematical learning disabilities: Rule or exception? The Open Rehabilitation Journal. 2008;**1**:15-16

[24] Lewis C, Hitch GJ, Walker P. The prevalence of specific arithmetic difficulties and specific reading difficulties in 9- to 10-year-old boys and girls. Journal of Child Psychology and Psychiatry. 1994;**35**:283-292. DOI: 10.1111/j.1469-7610.1994.tb01162.x

[25] Silva D, Colvin L, Glauert R, Stanley F, Srinivasjois R, Bower C. Literacy and numeracy underachievement in boys and girls with ADHD. Journal of Attention Disorders. 2015;**19**:1-12. DOI: 10.1177/1087054715596575

[26] Rubinsten O, Henik A. Developmental dyscalculia: Different mechanisms might not mean different mechanisms. Trends in Cognitive Sciences. 2009;**13**:92-99

[27] Piazza M. Neurocognitive start-up tools for symbolic number representations. Trends in Cognitive Sciences. 2010;**14**(12):542-551

[28] Dehaene S, Cohen L. Cultural recycling of cortical maps. Neuron. 2007;**56**(2):384-398. DOI: 10.1016/j.neuron.2007.10.004

[29] Piazza M, Izard V, Pinel P, Le Bihan D, Dehaene S. Tuning curves for approximate numerosity in the human intraparietal sulcus. Neuron. 2004;**44**(3):547-555. DOI: 10.1016/j.neuron.2004.10.014

[30] Feigenson L, Libertus ME, Halberda J. Links between the intuitive sense of number and formal mathematics ability. Child Development Perspectives. 2013;**7**(2):74-79. DOI: 10.1111/cdep.12019

[31] Gilmore CK, McCarthy SE, Spelke ES. Non-symbolic arithmetic abilities and mathematics achievement in the first year of formal schooling. Cognition. 2010;**115**(3):394-406. DOI: 10.1016/j.cognition.2010.02.002

[32] Halberda J, Mazzocco MMM, Feigenson L. Individual differences in non-verbal number acuity correlate with maths achievement. Nature. 2008;**455**(7213):665-668. DOI: 10.1038/nature07246

[33] Halberda J, Ly R, Wilmer JB, Naiman DQ, Germine L. Number sense across the lifespan as revealed by a massive Internet-based sample. Proceedings of the National Academy of Sciences of the United States of America. 2012;**109**(28):11116-11120. DOI: 10.1073/pnas.1200196109

[34] Libertus ME, Feigenson L, Halberda J. Preschool acuity of the approximate number system correlates with school math ability. Developmental Science. 2011;**14**(6):1292-1300. DOI: 10.1111/j.1467-7687.2011.01080.x

[35] Starr A, Libertus ME, Brannon EM. Number sense in infancy predicts mathematical abilities in childhood. Proceedings of the National Academy of Sciences of the United States of America. 2013;**110**(45):18116-18120. DOI: 10.1073/pnas.1302751110

[36] Starr A, DeWind NK, Brannon EM. The contributions of numerical acuity and non-numerical stimulus features to the development of the number sense and symbolic math achievement. Cognition. 2017;**168**:222-233. DOI: 10.1016/j.cognition.2017.07.004

[37] Starr A, Tomlinson RC, Brannon EM. The acuity and manipulability of the ANS have separable influences on preschoolers' symbolic math achievement. Frontiers in Psychology. 2018;**9**:2554. DOI: 10.3389/fpsyg.2018.02554

[38] Landerl K, Bevan A, Butterworth B. Developmental dyscalculia and basic numerical capacities: A study of 8-9-year-old students. Cognition. 2004;**93**(2):99-125. DOI: 10.1016/j.cognition.2003.11.004

[39] Mazzocco MMM, Feigenson L, Halberda J. Impaired acuity of the approximate number system underlies mathematical learning disability (dyscalculia). Child Development. 2011;**82**(4):1224-1237. DOI: 10.1111/j.1467-8624.2011.01608.x

[40] Sarnecka BW, Lee MD. Levels of number knowledge during early childhood. Journal of Experimental Child Psychology. 2009;**103**(3):325-337. DOI: 10.1016/j.jecp.2009.02.007

[41] Gallistel CR, Gelman R. Non-verbal numerical cognition: From reals to integers. Trends in Cognitive Sciences. 2000;**4**(2):59-65. DOI: 10.1016/S1364-6613(99)01424-2

[42] Krajewski K, Schneider W. Early development of quantity to number-word linkage as a precursor of mathematical school achievement and mathematical difficulties: Findings from a four-year longitudinal study. Learning and Instruction. 2009;**19**(6):513-526. DOI: 10.1016/j.learninstruc.2008.10.002

[43] Le Corre M, Carey S. One, two, three, four, nothing more: An investigation of the conceptual sources of the verbal counting principles. Cognition. 2007;**105**(2):395-438. DOI: 10.1016/j.cognition.2006.10.005

[44] Schneider M, Beeres K, Coban L, Merz S, Susan Schmidt S, Stricker J, et al. Associations of non-symbolic and symbolic numerical magnitude processing with mathematical competence: A meta-analysis. Developmental Science. 2017;**20**(3):e12372. DOI: 10.1111/desc.12372

[45] De Smedt B, Gilmore CK. Defective number module or impaired access? Numerical magnitude processing in first graders with mathematical difficulties. Journal of Experimental Child Psychology. 2011;**108**(2):278-292. DOI: 10.1016/j.jecp.2010.09.003

[46] De Smedt B, Noël MP, Gilmore C, Ansari D. How do symbolic and non-symbolic numerical magnitude processing skills relate to individual differences in children's mathematical skills? A review of evidence from brain and behavior. Trends in Neuroscience and Education. 2013;**2**:48-55. DOI: 10.1016/j.tine.2013.06.001

[47] Landerl K, Kölle C. Typical and atypical development of basic numerical skills in elementary school. Journal of Experimental Child Psychology. 2009;**103**(4):546-565. DOI: 10.1016/j.jecp.2008.12.006

[48] Simmons F, Singleton C, Horne J. Phonological awareness and visual-spatial sketchpad functioning predict early arithmetic attainment: Evidence from a longitudinal study. European Journal of Cognitive Psychology. 2008;**20**:711-722. DOI: 10.1080/09541440701614922

[49] Geary DC. From infancy to adulthood: The development of numerical abilities. European Child Adolescent Psychiatry. 2000;**2**(22):II11-II16. DOI: 10.1007/s007870070004

[50] Geary DC, Hoard MK, Hamson CO. Numerical and arithmetical cognition: Patterns of functions and deficits in children at risk for a mathematical disability. Journal of Experimental Child Psychology. 1999;**74**(3):213-239

[51] Geary DC, Hamson CO, Hoard MK. Numerical and arithmetical cognition: A longitudinal study of process and concept deficits in children with learning disability. Journal of Experimental Child Psychology. 2000;**77**(3):236-263

[52] Moura R, Wood G, Pinheiro-Chagas P, Lonnemann J, Krinzinger H, Willmes K, et al. Transcoding abilities in typical and atypical mathematics achievers: The role of working memory and procedural and lexical competencies. Journal of Experimental Child Psychology. 2013;**116**(3):707-727. DOI: 10.1016/j.jecp.2013.07.008

[53] Landerl K, Moll K. Comorbidity of learning disorders: Prevalence and familial transmission. Journal of Child Psychology and Psychiatry. 2010;**51**:287-294

[54] Simmons FR, Singleton C. Do weak phonological representations impact on arithmetic development? A review of research into arithmetic and dyslexia. Dyslexia. 2008;**14**(2):77-94. DOI: 10.1002/dys.341

[55] Currie J, Stabile M. Child mental health and human capital accumulation: The case of ADHD. Journal of Health Economics. 2006;**25**(6):1094-1118. DOI: 10.1016/j.jhealeco.2006.03.001

[56] Corbetta M, Shulman GL. Control of goal-directed and stimulus-driven attention in the brain. Nature Reviews Neuroscience. 2002;**3**(3):201-215. DOI: 10.1038/nrn755

[57] Goodale MA, Milner AD, Jakobson LS, Carey DP. A neurological dissociation between perceiving objects and grasping them. Nature. 1991;**349**(6305):154-156. DOI: 10.1038/349154a0

[58] Jung RE, Haier RJ. The parieto-frontal integration theory (P-FIT) of intelligence: Converging neuroimaging evidence. Behavioral and Brain Sciences. 2007;**30**(2):135-154. DOI: 10.1017/S0140525X07001185

[59] Ungerleider LG, Haxby JV. "What" and "where" in the human brain. Current Opinion in Neurobiology. 1994;**4**(2):157-165. DOI: 10.1016/0959-4388(94)90066-3

[60] Gilmore C, Attridge N, Clayton S, Cragg L, Johnson S, Marlow N, et al. Individual differences in inhibitory

control, not non-verbal number acuity, correlate with mathematics achievement. PLoS One. 2013;**8**(6):e67374. DOI: 10.1371/journal.pone.0067374

[61] Szucs D, Devine A, Soltesz F, Nobes A, Gabriel F. Developmental dyscalculia is related to visuo-spatial memory and inhibition impairment. Cortex. 2013;**49**(10):2674-2688. DOI: 10.1016/j.cortex.2013.06.007

[62] Moeller K, Pixner S, Zuber J, Kaufmann L, Nuerk HC. Early place-value understanding as a precursor for later arithmetic performance-A longitudinal study on numerical development. Research in Developmental Disabilities. 2011;**32**(5):1837-1851. DOI: 10.1016/j.ridd.2011.03.012

[63] Raghubar K, Cirino P, Barnes M, Ewing-Cobbs L, Fletcher J, Fuchs L. Errors in multi-digit arithmetic and behavioral inattention in children with math difficulties. Journal of Learning Disabilities. 2009;**42**:356-371. DOI: 10.1177/0022219409335211

[64] Cornoldi C, Mammarella I, Fine JG. Nonverbal Learning Disabilities. Oxford: Oxford University Press; 2016

[65] Drummond CR, Ahmad SA, Rourke BP. Rules for the classification of younger children with nonverbal learning disabilities and basic phonological processing disabilities. Archives of Clinical Neuropsychology. 2005;**20**(2):171-182. DOI: 10.1016/j.acn.2004.05.001

[66] Rourke BP, Conway JA. Disabilities of arithmetic and mathematical reasoning: Perspectives from neurology and neuropsychology. Journal of Learning Disabilities. 1997;**30**:34-46

[67] Bull R, Espy KA, Wiebe SA. Short-term memory, working memory, and executive functioning in preschoolers: Longitudinal predictors of mathematical achievement at age 7 years. Developmental Neuropsychology. 2008;**33**:205-228

[68] Geary DC. Mathematics and learning disabilities. Journal of Learning Disabilities. 2004;**37**:4-15

[69] Hitch GJ, McAuley E. Working memory in children with specific arithmetical learning difficulties. British Journal of Psychology. 1991;**82**(3):375-386. DOI: 10.1111/j.2044-8295.1991.tb02406.x

[70] Keeler ML, Swanson HL. Does strategy knowledge influence working memory in children with mathematical disabilities? Journal of Learning Disabilities. 2001;**34**(5):418-434. DOI: 10.1177/002221940103400504

[71] Passolunghi MC, Siegel LS. Short-term memory, working memory, and inhibitory control in children with difficulties in arithmetic problem solving. Journal of Experimental Child Psychology. 2001;**80**(1):44-57. DOI: 10.1006/jecp.2000.2626

[72] Passolunghi MC, Siegel LS. Working memory and access to numerical information in children with disability in mathematics. Journal of Experimental Child Psychology. 2004;**88**(4):348-367. DOI: 10.1016/j.jecp.2004.04.002

[73] Swanson HL. Cognitive processes that underlie mathematical precociousness in young children. Journal of Experimental Child Psychology. 2006;**93**:239-264

[74] Ashkenazi S, Rosenberg-Lee M, Tenison C, Menon V. Weak task-related modulation and stimulus representations during arithmetic problem solving in children with developmental dyscalculia. Developmental Cognitive Neuroscience.

2012;**2**(Suppl. 1):S152-S166. DOI: 10.1016/j.dcn.2011.09.006

[75] Noël MP, Turconi E. Assessing number transcoding in children. European Review of Applied Psychology. 1999;**49**(4):295-304

Chapter 9

Learning Disabilities in Children with Autism

Ingrid Ya I Sun, Ana Carolina Martins Cortez and Fernanda Dreux Miranda Fernandes

Abstract

Children with autism spectrum disorders often present signs of cognitive strategies that are not within the expected developmental profile. Therefore, it should be expected that the learning process of children with this disorder should be the focus of several studies regarding schooling and literacy. Unfortunately, that is not the real situation. In this chapter, the authors propose to present an overview of the available literature about learning, reading, and literacy in children with the autism spectrum disorders and report results of studies about the association between executive functions and reading abilities in children with autism spectrum disorders that attend to regular and special schools in Brazil.

Keywords: autism, children, language, learning, reading

1. Introduction

This chapter aims to gather and integrate studies on the development and neurocognitive processes involved in learning by children with autism spectrum disorder (ASD). It is believed that we need to know the neuropsychological foundations of learning for transmitting teaching.

Fonseca [1] describes that, although learning capacity is inherent to several species, the human is the only species that transmits teaching intentionally.

The literature reports that difficulties in learning conditional relationships between stimuli and concepts can lead to restrictions on an individual's life and limit their social interaction.

Communication plays an important role in integration of auditory and visual stimuli. This way, the understanding of the environment arises from the interaction between people, and learning is a result of the relationship created through sensory stimuli.

2. Learning by children with ASD: language, social, and cognitive factors

It is known that language occurs mostly by meaningful experiences and situations. Although it depends on cognitive development, physiological integrity, and linguistic abilities, the environmental demands and support have an essential role in the child's learning process. The construction of a socially shared code that leads to the assignment of meaning to the world's various elements and experiences depends on the interaction with other significant persons. Language and memory are also dependent on meaningful situations and experiences. Abilities acquired through systematic training, despite frequently presenting fast results, are discarded as fast as they are acquired if they are not used or associated with meaningful contexts.

Based on these ideas, it seems reasonable to suppose that children with autism spectrum disorders present some disadvantage in the learning process because they have a social inability that is inherent to the ASD features, with varied degrees of impairment in social interactions. This way, it is accepted that language impairment of children with autism is not necessarily associated with linguistic structures, although they are affected in some children. Language impairments of children with ASD are essentially related to pragmatic abilities, also involving different levels of inabilities, from the lack of contact to subtle difficulties regarding interaction and conversation abilities. This is another reason why it is fundamental to understand the child's context and environment, to assess the impact of each child's inabilities and design intervention plans that address the most efficient and timely intervention.

Several recent studies show that including families in the therapeutic process of children with ASD increases better outcomes and prognosis than traditional one-on-one therapeutic approaches.

Authors like Winnicot [2] consider emotional health as the development's "back bone," allowing cognitive and linguistic development and therefore enabling successful learning processes. Regardless of the causal relation and of the hierarchy among these areas of development, the importance of emotional health to learning is unquestionable. Perceiving and processing sensorial information and positively assimilating and interpreting information in order to build and learn healthily and creatively—that is, so that cognitive processing really occurs—depend on emotional health.

Studies that focus on the importance of engaging parents and caregivers are increasing in number and impact, with results increasingly consistent showing that the quality of life of parents and caregivers as well as their involvement in the intervention processes with children with ASD has a positive influence in the outcomes of these processes.

The symptoms often found that ASD individuals also fit in the attention deficit hyperactivity disorder (ADHD) diagnosis, leading researches to compare learning performance between individuals with ASD and ADHD. Both diagnoses present significant impairments in cognitive performance, and it is important to make considerations from the neurocognitive perspective, raising questions and studies that involve tasks that require skills such as executive function (EF), theory of mind (ToM), language, and even correlations between them, seeking possible relations of causality.

EF is currently defined as a cognitive process necessary to define a goal and accomplish it, including the skills needed for it. Among them, working memory, inhibitory control, and cognitive flexibility are included. Working memory is the ability to rescue information previously stored to accomplish a task. Inhibitory control is the ability to suppress any actions or information that may interrupt or hinder the execution of the task or planning.

EF is closely linked to communicative skills, impacting learning, autonomy, and social life of the individual with ASD. This, in part, makes it difficult to understand the direct impact of EF impairment on children with ASD. Even the studies do not yet reach a consensus on impairments in EF in this population. Some studies indicate deficit and risk indicating the causal relationship between EF and other abilities, while others show that individuals with ASD do not present greater impairment than other groups with typical development (TD), developmental language disorder (DLD), and ADHD, indicating that this may not be the central impairment of the disorder.

Some researchers, including Kado and collaborators [3], report in their paper that the working memory performance of children with ASD and ADHD is similar, but their performance is below when compared with TD children, even when matched with IQ and school age. However, other researchers like Roleofs and collaborators did not find significant differences in working memory between adolescents and adults with ASD and intellectual disability when compared with individuals without ASD matched with IQ [4]. In an attempt to understand the interdependence of working memory with language, some studies separate the assessment of this cognitive ability between visual or spatial working memory and verbal working memory. A very interesting research that tries to understand the relation of working memory and language ability was Hill's paper in 2015 [5]. The working memory was evaluated and compared in 5- to 8-year-old children with ASD and DLD. In this study, children with ASD were separated into two groups: children with and without language impairment. Children with proper language had better performances than children with language impairment. In addition, children with ASD and impaired language performed similarly to children with DLD in most verbal working memory tasks, but none of these groups differed in visual working memory tasks, suggesting their interdependence. This also happens with inhibition control.

The findings of inhibitory control studies in children with ASD are diverse. Some indicate significant losses, while others find no differences compared to ADHD and DT. A widely used test to verify this ability is Stroop, which requires a refined language skill. Corbett and his collaborators [6] performed several inhibitory control tests, with and without the need for verbal expressive language. In the test, requiring verbal ability, children with ASD and ADHD had worse performances than TD children. In the test where the verbal expressive ability was not required—children should heard or saw a certain number to answer or not—children with ASD performed worse than children with DT and ADHD. However, it is important to note that, even in the test of visual working memory, which supposed to not requiring expressive language, the task required a linguistic ability.

And the same pattern happens in researches that attempt to assess cognitive flexibility [7] using tasks that require some level of language, comprehensive or expressive.

The fact that neuropsychological assessments are intended to assess language and are not sensitive to these skills has been a frequent problem in most proposed assessments. In general, these assessments are made by psychologists who don't have deep knowledge to determine language failures or even to distinguish or define the language structures required for that. Many misjudge language only as an expressive or verbal act, which is conceptually wrong, or disregard the cultural component of language, or even fail to evaluate language ability alone, often considering the cognitive strategies used by the child as language ability or otherwise. And as noted above, this knowledge is essential to clarify a possible causal relationship or to shed light on the possible association between cognitive and language areas, not only in children with ASD.

3. Learning to read

For children with typical development, learning to speak can naturally come out observing and participating in moments and situations of communication with their parents and their community.

In contrast, the act of learning to read and write is a complex task, composed of multiple interdependent processes, including understanding how the visual symbols correspond to spoken language [8].

There is a range of articles that discuss the importance and interdependence of good oral language development for the success of written code acquisition, since writing is considered a representation of language.

The literature of clinical neuropsychology reports that an assessment of cognitive strengths and weaknesses is useful for children with any developmental or learning disorder [9]. Considering the heterogeneity of the clinical settings of children with ASD, assessing and understanding the child's individual strengths and weaknesses help better focus school plans and medical treatment and understand the possible areas of difficulty [9, 10].

Westerveld et al. [11] argue that learning to read is just another challenge for children with ASD. In their study, they found that approximately 30–60% of these children present some difficulty to develop literacy. It is important to highlight that even higher functioning children are also part of the statistics.

Jones et al. [12] described that the cognitive heterogeneity of children with ASD is an element that makes it difficult to characterize the academic difficulties of this population. In addition, they report that cognitive abilities may not be congruent with their writing operations.

In their paper, Fletcher and Miciak [9] argue the fact that some children have deficits in cognitive tests may not necessarily indicate causal direction in a child's learning difficulties. A cognitive deficit does not indicate "why" a child has a learning problem.

Another possible justification found in the literature for this variation in the development of reading and writing in children with ASD is the individual differences in language skills in the areas of phonology, semantics, and syntax [11, 12].

Davidson and Weismer [10] describe that reading disabilities can be classified based on problems that arise in decoding or comprehension abilities. It's important to know the history of reading instruction for children with exceptional educational needs to consider what is known about reading abilities in individuals with ASD [13].

Gabig [14] in her study with children with ASD, who reduced performance in areas such as vocabulary, may have negative influences on skills such as phonological processing. In addition, she found that some abilities related to decoding ability appear to be relatively intact.

Richardson and Heikki [8] discuss that the reasons for the phonological deficit in autism are still not clear but certainly interfere in the quality of mental representations and in the quality of the lexical, creating a poor link between the phonological awareness and reading skills.

Other authors question whether insufficient performance in reading skills are from specific verbal material defects or the consequence of perceptual, temporal, or long-term memory failure problems [15].

Overall, studies indicate that although the ability to recognize written words may be similar to that of typically developing learners, children with ASD tend to have deficits in integrating information. That is, they have difficulty retrieving and integrating meanings necessary for reading comprehension, including the ability to create connections between content read with prior knowledge and the ability to make inferences [16].

The literature describes that most children with autism show average ability to recognize words while reading and to accurately spell words for age and grade level. In contrast, what the literature cannot yet explain is whether phonological awareness accompanies the good performance of phonetic decoding presented by children with autism [14].

There are several studies that speculate if children with ASD would perform poorer when decoding pseudowords than when reading sight words because of a rote memorization of the visual shape of words. Most of their results indicated that children with autism do not show preference for the visual recognition of sight words over the decoding of pseudowords. It suggests that ASD children are capable of using visual and phonological recognition process to identify written words. Thus, studies lead us to believe that children with autism can benefit from other access channels to achieve good reading and writing performance.

Hyperlexia is frequently one condition presented by children with ASD. It is characterized by a child's precocious ability to read (far above what would be expected at their age). As with all individuals, children with hyperlexia have a wide range of skills and deficits. The high abilities to decode do not exclude the possibility that children may have a cognitive, language learning and/or social disorder.

What experts argue is that content that can be "formally" taught can be more easily learned by children with ASD. Already "intuitive" content such as phonological awareness skills would be less understood by this population.

Corso et al. [17] tested the correlation between reading tasks and different neuropsychological functions. They concluded that the strongest significant correlations occurred during executive functions tasks.

Pellicano [18] pointed out that there are no studies that explicitly investigate the nature of executive functions in autism, arguing that there are only researches with the fractionation of these functions, that is, as if just one of these components can be specifically affected in autism.

It is also often possible to find studies that compare the performance of children with ASD in theory of mind abilities (ToM). Some studies report that children with executive function deficits but with intact theory of mind abilities are hardly found.

Since the use of theory of mind abilities is essential to the mental and behavioral functioning, understanding the nature of these skills cannot be discarded during the assessment of reading and writing skills [19].

One of the reasons why individuals with ASD may have difficulties in representing situations involving theory of mind may be explained by the fact that they have difficulty integrating clues that are relevant to the context and self-representation.

This would be a justification for the text comprehension difficulties so often observed in this population, especially the difficulties related to understanding pragmatic and nonliteral aspects of language.

Deficits in the functioning of EF and literacy may differ between disturbances. Assessing them and identifying their deficits can provide information on which systems may be impaired and, most importantly, what can be done to stimulate them.

4. Important considerations for clinical intervention in SLP

The intervention approach may consider all areas of oral or written language where the children have deficits. It's important to associate information about the student's facilitating routes, whether auditory, visual, or motor. This way, the therapist should investigate whether the influence of several processing modalities obtain a more comprehensive understanding of the child's potential perceptual abilities.

Bosseler and Massaro [20] describe that technology is also being used in educational settings as an effective method of getting children engaged.

Some authors argue that if we guarantee the use of materials that address the different routes, learning can occur simply due to multiple exposures without necessarily having feedback and formal interference from the therapist. Although Bosseler and Massaro observed that children profited from seeing and hearing, spoken language can better guide language learning than modality alone.

What we should expect is that stimulated content must be learned operatively, processed, stored, and related to a set of experience to apply functionality and use it in a meaningful way.

Currently, there are already some available therapeutic methods that can be developed by parents at home. However, there are not yet numerous clinical articles that allow a more accurate interpretation of the results. Thus, there are limitations in measuring the effectiveness of these approaches in treating autistic children, especially in the long-term.

There are authors who emphasize how important it is to encourage these types of family-based therapeutic approaches as key interveners; however, understand that caregiver training should be done very carefully so that such interventions are not inadequately developed and reinforce difficulties and changes in child development.

5. Conclusion

As we have seen, environmental support plays an essential role in the child's learning process. The findings suggest that children with autism spectrum disorders (ASD) have some disadvantage in the learning process due to their inherent social disability to ASD characteristics.

The literature describes that parental support and engagement in intervention processes with children with ASD positively influence the outcomes of these processes. Therefore, the intervention process should encompass all the possibilities and resources of oral and written language stimulation, associated with the information and collaboration presented by the caregivers.

The learning disabilities of children with autism exist, and our ultimate goal for these children is to create a connection between learning and functionality.

Author details

Ingrid Ya I Sun*, Ana Carolina Martins Cortez
and Fernanda Dreux Miranda Fernandes
School of Medicine of University of Sao Paulo, São Paulo, Brazil

*Address all correspondence to: ya.ingrid@gmail.com

References

[1] Fonseca V. Papel das funções cognitivas, conotativas e executivas na aprendizagem: uma abordagem neuropsicológica. Revista da Associação Brasileira de Psicopedagogia. 2014;**31**(96):236-253

[2] Winnicott DW. Playing and Reality. London: Tavistock; 1971

[3] Kado Y, Sanada S, Yanagihara M, et al. Executive function in children with pervasive developmental disorder and attention-deficit/hyperactivity disorder assessed by the Keio version of the Wisconsin card sorting test. Brain & Development. 2012;**34**(05):354-359

[4] Roleofs RL, Visser EM, Berger HJC, Prins JB, Van Schrojenstein Lantman-De Valk HMJ, Teunisse JP. Executive functioning in individuals with intellectual disabilities and autism spectrum disorders. Journal of Intellectual Disability Research. 2015;**59**(02):125-137

[5] Hill AP, Van Santen J, Gorman K, Laghorst BH, Fombonne E. Memory in language-impaired children with and without autism. Journal of Neurodevelopmental Disorder. 2015;**7**(01):10

[6] CorbettBA, ConstantineLJ, HendrenR, Rocke D, Ozonoff S. Examining executive functioning in children with autism spectrum disorder, attention deficit hyperactivity disorder and typical development. Psychiatry Research. 2009;**166**(2-3):210-222

[7] Leung RC, Zakanis KK. Brief report: Cognitive flexibility in autism spectrum disorders: A quantitative review. Journal of Autism & Developmental Disorders. 2014;**44**(10):2628-2645

[8] Richardson U, Lyytinen H. The GraphoGame method: The theoretical and methodological background of the technology-enhanced learning environment for learning to read. Human Technology. 2014;**10**(1):39-60. DOI: 10.17011/ht/urn.201405281859

[9] Fletcher JM, Jeremy M. Comprehensive cognitive assessments are not necessary for the identification and treatment of learning disabilities. Archives of Clinical Neuropsychology. 2017;**32**(1):2-7. DOI: 10.1093/arclin/acw103

[10] Davidson MM, Weismer SL. Characterization and prediction of early reading abilities in children on the autism spectrum. Journal of Autism & Developmental Disorders. 2014;**44**(4):828-845. DOI: 10.1007/s10803-013-1936-2

[11] Westerveld MF et al. A systematic review of the literature on emergent literacy skills of preschool children with autism spectrum disorder. The Journal of Special Education. 2016;**50**(1):37-48. DOI: 10.1177/0022466915613593

[12] Jones CRG, Happé F, Golden H, Marsden AJS, Tregay J, Simonoff E, et al. Reading and arithmetic in adolescents with autism spectrum disorders: Peaks and dips in attainment. Neuropsychology. 2009;**23**(6):718-728. DOI: 10.1037/a0016360

[13] Brown HM, Oram-Cardy J, Johnson A. A meta-analysis of the reading comprehension skills of individuals on the autism spectrum. Journal of Autism and Developmental Disorders. 2013;**43**(4):932-955. DOI: 10.1007/s10803-012-1638-1

[14] Gabig CS. Phonological awareness and word recognition in reading by children with autism. Communication Disorders Quarterly. 2010. DOI: 10.1177/1525740108328410

[15] Capovilla AGS, Joly MCRA, Ferracini F, Caparrotti NB, Carvalho MR, Raad AJ. Estratégias de leitura e desempenho em escrita no início da alfabetização. Psicologia Escolar e Educacional. 2004;**8**(2):189-197. DOI: 10.1590/S1413-85572004000200007

[16] Nunes DRP, Walter EC. Processos de leitura em educandos com autismo: um estudo de revisão. Revista Brasileira de Educação Especial, Marília;**22, 2016**(4):619-632

[17] Corso HV, Sperb TM, Jou GI, Salles JF. Metacognição e funções executivas: relações entre os conceitos e implicações para a aprendizagem. Psicologia: Teoria e Pesquisa. 2013;**29**(1):21-29. DOI: 10.1590/S0102-37722013000100004

[18] Pellicano E. Links between theory of mind and executive function in young children with autism: Clues to developmental primacy. Developmental Psychology. 2007;**43**(4):974-990. DOI: 10.1037/0012 1649.43.4.974

[19] Meyer LKC. A Compreensão de leitura e a Teoria da Mente em crianças com autismo. Pouso Alegre. 2018:190f

[20] Massaro DW, Bosseler A. Read my lips: The importance of the face in a computer-animated tutor for vocabulary learning by children with autism. Autism. 2006;**10**(5):495-510. DOI: 10.1177/1362361306066599

Section 4

Assessment of Speech and Language-Based Learning Disabilities

Chapter 10

Contradictions around Inter-collegial Collaboration Regarding Differentiated Assessment for Pupils with Dyslexia in Greek State Secondary Schools

Maria Rontou

Abstract

This chapter discusses the issue of inter-collegial collaboration regarding differentiated assessment and marking for students with dyslexia in two Greek state secondary schools. Activity theory is used to analyse the contradictions that arise around the issue of differentiated assessment for pupils with dyslexia from data collected from interviews with headteachers, teachers, pupils and parents and field notes from observation across two schools. The analysis demonstrates that contradictions are created when participants try to achieve their goals for differentiation by the lack of staff meetings and collaboration between colleagues in the same school. The findings suggest the necessity of a staff meeting in the beginning of the school year regarding students with dyslexia requiring support and differentiation or the introduction of a list of pupils with dyslexia and their profiles.

Keywords: pupils with dyslexia, inter-collegial collaboration, differentiated assessment, contradictions, secondary schools

1. Introduction

This chapter discusses the issue of inter-collegial collaboration regarding differentiated assessment and marking for students with dyslexia in two Greek state secondary schools. Collaboration between colleagues is necessary for dyslexia provision. Mackay suggests that portraits on all pupils with specific learning difficulties including individual teaching and learning strategies should be available to all staff [1]. The introduction of student profiles was an example of a successful initiative taken by SENCOs in Hunter-Carsch study [2]. SEN directories and student profiles were introduced in one school in order to increase the effectiveness of communication between SEN staff and curriculum subject teachers. Pollock and Waller also mention the difficulty of special needs teachers to communicate with all subject teachers about individual students [3]. They suggest that a list of pupils requiring support circulates regularly emphasizing their particular needs. They also suggest that all teachers communicate regarding students with dyslexia.

As far as the Greek context is concerned, Arapogianni reported lack of contact and collaboration of teachers with other professionals [4]. Lappas also reported lack of communication and collaboration between learning support teachers and mainstream teachers in Greek primary schools because of the lack of responsibility of the headteachers for the provision for specific learning difficulties, which lay only with the learning support teachers [5]. In my study, I used similar methods (semi-structured interviews) to investigate if inter-collegial communication is effective from the perspective of parents, pupils and teachers and headteachers but not learning support teachers and policy agents as Lappas [5] did. Furthermore, my study was carried out in secondary schools as opposed to primary schools in Lappas [5].

1.1 Theoretical framework

A theoretical framework was needed for this study that explores human learning within organizational systems in a collective way. Activity theory and the work of Engestrom provided one such framework [6]. Sociocultural activity theory was initiated by Vygotsky when he tried to explain the learning process by arguing that learning enables people to think or do something beyond their capability and this is done in a historical, cultural and social context, with one or more people [7, 8]. Vygotsky believed that human activity happens when the subjects, those whose actions are analysed, resolve a shared problem, an 'object', by using 'tools' to achieve a goal [9]. Engeström [6] describes how the current understanding of activity theory has evolved through three generations of research. The first generation contributed to activity theory the idea of 'mediation', which was represented in Vygotsky's [8] triangular model (**Figure 1**) linking the subject and the object through mediating artefacts [6].

In the second generation, which was developed from Leont'ev's writing [6, 10, 11], Engeström expanded the triangular representation of an activity system to enable the examination of activity systems at an organizational level as opposed to a focus on the individual actors operating with tools [12]. This expansion of the Vygotskian triangle represents the social or organizational elements in an activity system through the addition of the elements of community, rules and division of labour (see **Figure 2**).

Activity theory was selected as a theoretical framework for the data collection and analysis of this study because it allowed the inclusion of different groups of participants and the investigation of the relationship between them. The second principle of activity theory, multi-voicedness, was useful for this study as it allowed the investigation of multiple points of view on the same issue, that of the EFL teachers, the students, the parents and the Ministry of Education [6].

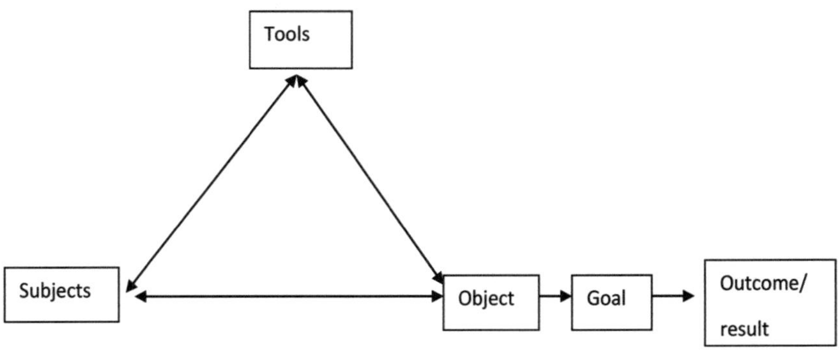

Figure 1.
The principal relationship in an activity system.

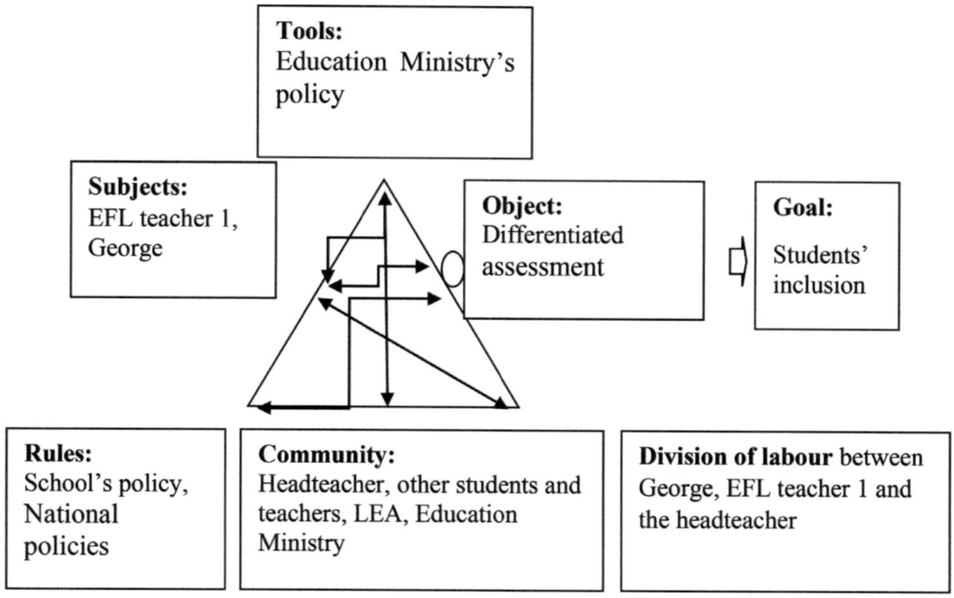

Figure 2.
Second generation of activity theory.

Therefore, the subjects of learning of the activity system in School 1, the school where the study took place, are English as a Foreign Language (EFL) teacher 1 and one student with dyslexia, George (see **Figure 2**). A possible object of learning, that is, what the subjects are working on, is differentiated assessment [12]. The goal in an activity system is the result of the 'creative effort' that can be met when the problems are resolved [13]. A possible goal in this study is the inclusion of students with dyslexia.

The community representing the wider sociocultural influences includes the context of the activity, that is, the people who are concerned with the same object: the headteacher of the school, the other students and teachers, the Local Education Authority (LEA) and the Ministry of Education [12, 14]. Therefore, the activity is a collective one and not an individual action of the teacher only or the students only [6].

The division of labour in this study refers to the division of tasks between the EFL teacher, the headteacher and student. The rules are the principles regulating the actions of the participants and they can be both written and unwritten, for example, the national policies on dyslexia and their interpretations by the headteacher of the school as well as the routines and professional practices of the teachers [12].

Since activity theory is deeply contextual and studies specific local practices, it is often linked with the use of case study (e.g. [6, 15, 16]) that takes context and its details into account [17]. An appropriate design for this study using activity theory as a theoretical framework was a case study. A case study was suitable for this study as it aimed to go into sufficient detail and explore the complexities of dyslexia provision and multiple sources were necessary for the collection of data [17].

1.2 Methodology

1.2.1 Methods

The study included multiple methods for triangulation purposes, which is a characteristic of case studies [18]: semi-structured and unstructured ethnographic interviews with two EFL teachers, one teacher of Greek, two headteachers, one student with dyslexia and his parents and lesson observation with field notes and digital audio recording of EFL lessons.

The interviews with participants were carried out in the Greek language and they were transcribed and were translated into English. This process involved construction of meaning and interpretations by the transcriber and translator [19]. One problem was that the interviews were in spoken form transcribed in the Greek language, which had to be translated in written form in the English language. This created a problem of equivalence.

The case studies in this paper are ethnographic because this study had a longitudinal element as it included the researcher's contact with the participants in schools and their houses over a long period of time [20]. The researcher spent 13 weeks collecting data with School 1 participants and 16 weeks collecting data with School 2 participants. The researcher also kept contact with EFL teacher 2 and attended seminars with her the year after the study.

The data were analysed using activity theory in order to investigate the perspective of the different groups of participants and the relationship between them as well as the relationship between the participants and the tools, the rules, the community and the division of labour and how these influence the achievement of participants' goals. The analysis focused on patterns in teachers', students' and parents' needs as well as on the contradictions in the achievement of the participants' goals. Contradictions are tensions or dilemmas that arise from the processes within and between the elements of the activity system and become the object of collaborative learning [9]. Therefore, the aim of the analysis is to identify the contradictions that appear when the teachers, students and parents try to work on their objects as well as the factors that created these contradictions. Contradictions between elements of the activity system are indicated in the figures by lightning-shaped arrows [16].

1.2.2 Context and participants

The data for this study come from two state secondary schools in Athens, School 1 and School 2. School 1 was an upper secondary school while School 2 was a lower secondary school. The data used in this paper from School 1 involved an EFL teacher, a headteacher, a student with dyslexia, George and his parents. George was 17 years old and attended the second year of senior high school. He was diagnosed with dyslexia at the age of 14. He attended EFL lessons up to B class at a language school. EFL teacher 1 had 19 years of teaching experience, 6 out of which were at the state sector. The data used in this chapter from School 2 involved an EFL teacher and a headteacher. EFL teacher 2 had 19 years of teaching experience, 8 of which were at the state sector.

The selection of schools was guided by convenience, that is, the accessibility of schools and the availability of individuals in them due to professional contacts [21, 22]. The researcher was also informed by the headteacher that there were students with dyslexia in the school. The EFL teachers that participated in the study were teachers who had pupils with dyslexia in their classes and who agreed to participate in the study after being informed about its aims and procedure.

The criterion for choosing students was a dyslexia diagnosis and their parents' informed consent to participate in the study. In order not to identify the school and the participants, pseudonyms were used for the students and the teachers' names were replaced with codes like EFL teacher 2, headteacher 2, mother 1 and father 1 [23].

The researcher was not a teacher at the schools in which the research was conducted but was a teacher permanently employed by the Greek Ministry of Education working in another LEA. Although she was not an employee in the two schools, the researcher was part of the same culture, had gone through the same educational system, had grown up and went to school in the same area as the first school and had lived in the area of the second school.

2. Findings

2.1 The parents' perspective in School 1

I next investigate whether teachers in School 1 collaborate with each other for dyslexia issues. I explore the issue from the perspective of the parents, the student, the headteacher, the EFL teacher and the teacher of Greek of School 1.

George's parents were especially unhappy with the lack of information to teachers about the students with dyslexia in their classes. George's father complained that when he went to the school the year before the research was carried out to talk to the teachers, he was told that George had not informed teachers about his 'diagnosis' (Extract 1):

Extract 1. Interview with George's parents.

F1 ... last year was his worst year at school
M it was the worst yes
F1 he felt ... something with the teachers, I had gone two or three times. When I tell [teachers] 'he has [dyslexia]', 'he hasn't told me' eh how hasn't he told you? If George is expelled for five days don't teachers tell each other? That is don't you notice this problem?
M teachers don't collaborate with each other
F1 yes this is my problem, that is, I went nuts last year.

Furthermore, George's father felt disappointed the year before the study took place when he saw that George's diagnosis was the first on the pile when the teacher of Greek opened the folder in front of him:

Extract 2. Interview with George's parents.

F1 ... and last year when the teacher of Greek opened the folder the paper [diagnosis] that we had taken that he has a problem was on top so how come they not know?

As a result of not being informed, some teachers refused to differentiate testing for George, for example, they refused to examine him orally:

Extract 3. Interview with George's parents.

Mo1 not only did they not know that there was a problem that is, ... when we went George was finishing the first four months and they hadn't even gone to the trouble of telling him 'come to tell us [the answers] orally'

Last year, the history teacher refused to examine George orally and the same happened this year also with the theoretical subjects of Principle of Economic Theory and Principles of Management and Administration of Business and Services:

Extract 4. Interview with George's parents.

F1 Last year while he was writing history and he says 'can I say it orally?' because George will make a mistake, 'it doesn't matter George', she says, why doesn't it matter?
Mo1 It doesn't matt- George she says, 'instead of 18 you get 15', 'why did I get 15?' 'Because there is no clear meaning'... 'I can tell you orally', 'eh now [how can we do it]
M When did this happen?
Mo1 Now now, this has happened now as well
M With teachers of Greek?
Mo1 I can't remember if it happened with a teacher of Greek, it has happened with a theoretical subject that you could say it orally that is. In economics and in business management it has happened sometime.

George's and his parents' object in the activity system in **Figure 3** during the year before the research was carried out was to inform George's teachers about his diagnosis. Their goal was to make sure teachers differentiated their teaching and assessment for George. The teachers are not in the subject position as I cannot know if they wanted to be informed or not considering at least two of them were not willing to examine George orally. There was a contradiction in the teachers' not being informed about and not using the tool of George's diagnostic report, which made the object and the goal difficult to meet. This contradiction could have been resolved by either the parents going to the school at the end of the first 4-month period or the student telling the teachers about his diagnosis after getting his exam result. The goal of differentiated assessment and marking was not achieved with the history teacher last year even after she was informed about his diagnosis by George (Extract 4).

2.2 George's perspective for the current year

Because of his past year's experiences, George decided to inform the teachers of the subjects for which he would have to take exams for entering university about his dyslexia from the beginning of this school year as he wanted to be given good grades in these subjects (Extract 5, lines 340–341). It is interesting though that George informed only the specialization subject teachers about his dyslexia and not the general education subject teachers such as the EFL teacher and a teacher of Greek whom I interviewed because he did not care about these subjects. His parents also mentioned this (Extract 5, lines 336–337).

However, it seems that last year's situation is being repeated this year as two teachers, the teachers of Development of Applications in Programming and Principles of Management and Administration of Business and Services, have refused to examine George orally or at least to differentiate their marking in exams although they were told that he had difficulty expressing his thoughts in written form and he wanted to be examined orally (Extract 5).

Extract 5. Interview with George's parents.

332 M But he went and told them himself in specialization subjects
333 Mo1 In specialization
334 M Teachers of the rest of the subjects didn't know
335 Mo1 Yes yes yes
336 F1 But he doesn't care
337 Mo1 We said this that he doesn't care at all for the general education subjects
338 but where he cared ... he went alone

339 M Ah he went
340 Mo1 And he said from the start 'I have dysgrafia, I want you to pay attention
341 to it'

The activity system of School 1 in terms of George's object for the current year (informed specialization teachers) is presented in **Figure 4**. Second generation of activity theory [6] is applied to analyse this theme as both George and his current teachers belong to the same institution and the same community with the same rules. George's object was to be taught by specialization teachers who were informed about his dyslexia and differentiate his assessment and marking of his paper. He knew from previous experience that his specialization subjects' teachers would not be informed about his dyslexia in the beginning of the year. For this reason, he informed them about it although it was not his responsibility to do so. George's behaviour was innovative; he tried to solve the problem in the activity system on his own, subverting the rules of the activity system of School 1, the usual practices that require the headteacher to inform teachers about students' diagnoses rather than the students themselves. George's innovative behaviour led to the partial achievement of his goal, which was differentiation in assessment and marking, as two teachers still refused to differentiate their marking. I showed that George's parents and George would have liked to have informed teachers on students' diagnoses in order to have the provision he deserves but this was not always the case.

2.3 Professionals' perspectives in School 1

I next explore whether headteacher 1 informed teachers about the students with dyslexia in School 1 and how a teacher from the lower secondary school informed EFL teacher 2 from the upper secondary school (School 1).

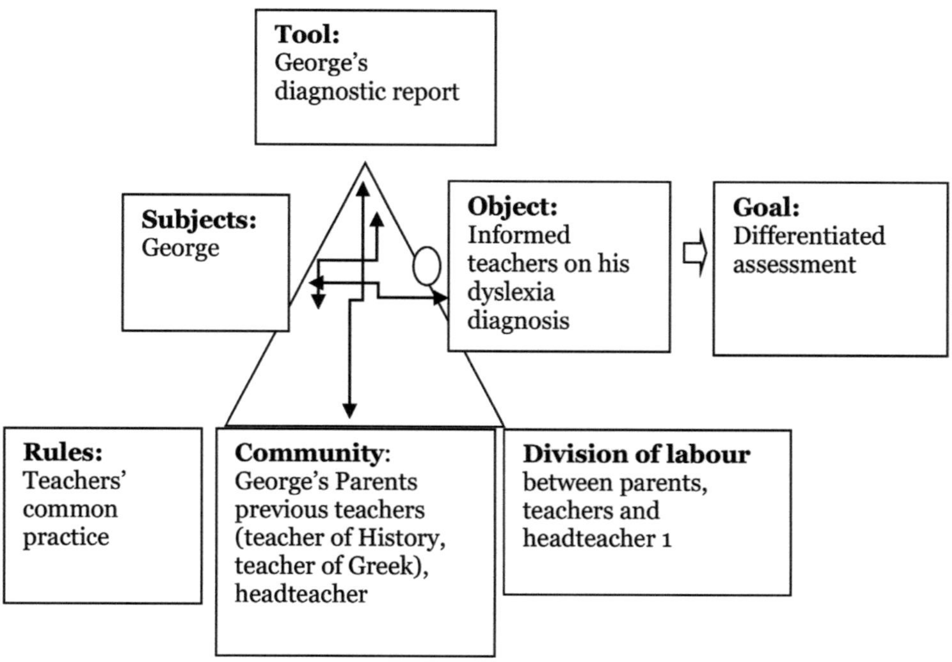

Figure 3.
George's object and goal for previous year.

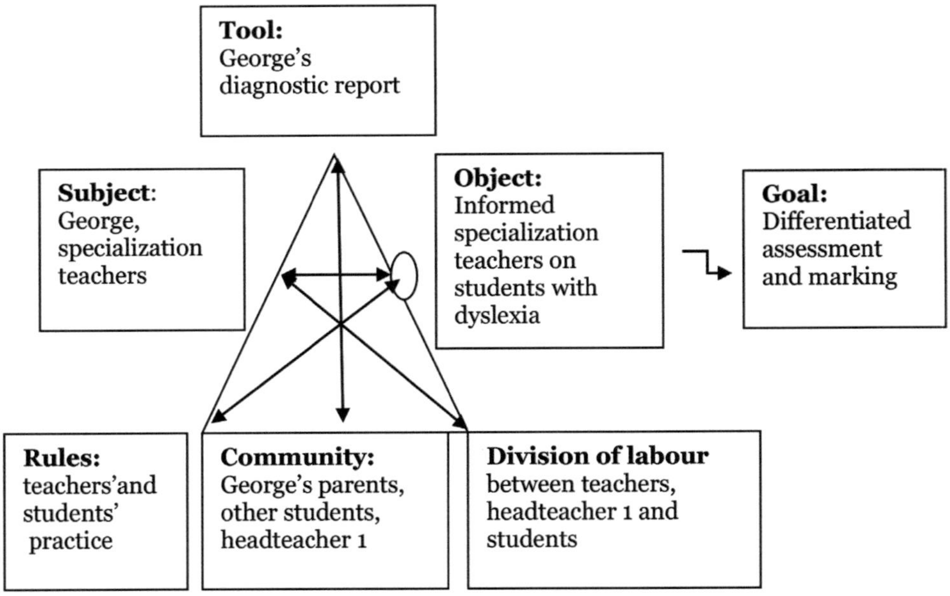

Figure 4.
Informed specialization teachers.

When I started the study in School 1, the headteacher told me that the teachers who have students with dyslexia in their classes are always informed about the students with dyslexia and the children are supported:

Extract 6. Interview with HT1.

> *M Have all the teachers been informed?*
> *HT1 Yes, always when a student comes, when such a student exists the teachers who teach the specific class are informed and this child is helped because of this problem*

This interview gave me the impression that the headteacher talked generally about what is done in schools regarding dyslexia, not what happened in his school. I came to this conclusion because when I met the EFL teacher a month earlier she was not informed by the headteacher about this issue but by a teacher of Greek from the lower secondary school in the same building. This is what I wrote in my field notes about this:

Extract 7. Field notes.

> *She [the EFL teacher] wasn't informed by the headteacher about the fact that these students have dyslexia because both she and the headteacher came to the school this year. A teacher of Greek from the lower secondary school told her about these students because she had taught them at lower secondary school.*

At an organizational level, there is no collaborative mechanism between the lower secondary and upper secondary school to exchange information on students with dyslexia. At an individual level, the teacher of Greek from the lower secondary school (subjects, **Figure 5**) gave information on the student with dyslexia (George) to the EFL teacher in the upper secondary school in order to facilitate my study. She gave the information that the EFL teacher (subject) needed to receive in order to differentiate her teaching. In this way, she subverted the rules of professional practice, which require that the headteacher informs teachers about students with dyslexia (contradiction). The teacher of Greek offered the EFL teacher a 'what artifact' that she could use to achieve the goal of differentiated teaching.

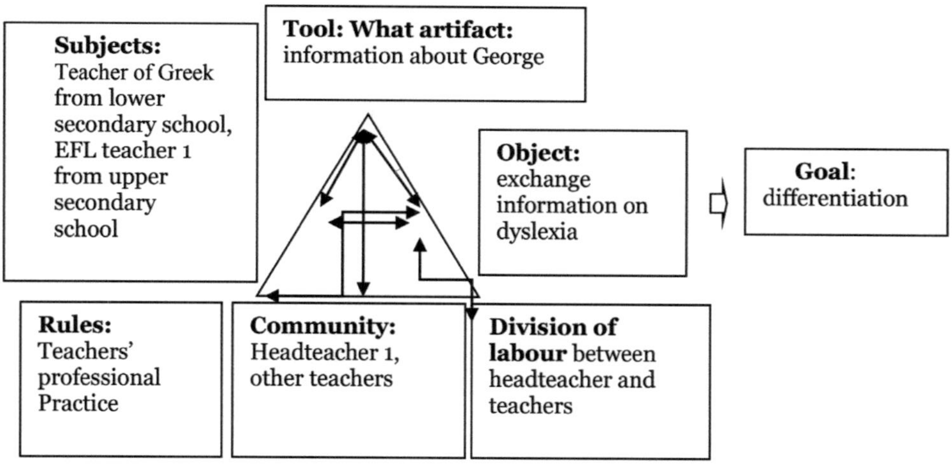

Figure 5.
Teacher of Greek and EFL teacher 1 exchanging information.

This artefact influenced the community in School 1, that is, the headteacher and possibly other teachers in School 1. When my research started, the teacher of Greek from the lower secondary school informed EFL teacher 1. EFL teacher 1 probably searched for students' diagnostic reports. She must have asked the headteacher to give her the reports or tell her who the students with dyslexia were since she mentioned to me the other two students with a diagnosis of dyslexia during the study. She mentioned a boy in January (*there is another boy who is supposed to have [dyslexia]...* Interview with T1) and a girl in February:

Extract 8. Interview with T1.

> *T1 ... there are students like I said, a female student there is in the other class, who, while she has a paper [diagnosis], I don't see her facing this problem.*

When I talked to the teacher of Greek of George's class in December she was not aware of George's diagnosis of dyslexia either:

Extract 9. Field notes.

> *She [the teacher of Greek] didn't know that George had a diagnosis, she hasn't seen his writing yet as they haven't written an exam yet and it is the first year that she teaches his class. She didn't happen to see his file with his report either.*

This suggests that in the beginning of the year there was no appropriate staff meeting or no other effective way of informing teachers on students with dyslexia.

When I asked the EFL teacher later during the study, in January, if she collaborates with the headteacher about dyslexia issues, she said that she does in order for the headteacher to inform her about students with dyslexia. However, he does not tell her how to examine them because he probably does not know either:

Extract 10. Interview with teacher 1.

> *M Do you collaborate with the headteacher?*
> *T1 Look... I collaborate so that they tell me first of all who they are ...*
> *M Has he told you what to do in exams?*
> *T1 No there isn't such a thing, because who knows? Who knows?*

In **Figure 6**, the activity system of School 1 is presented. The learning object for EFL teacher 1 and the teacher of Greek is to receive information on students with

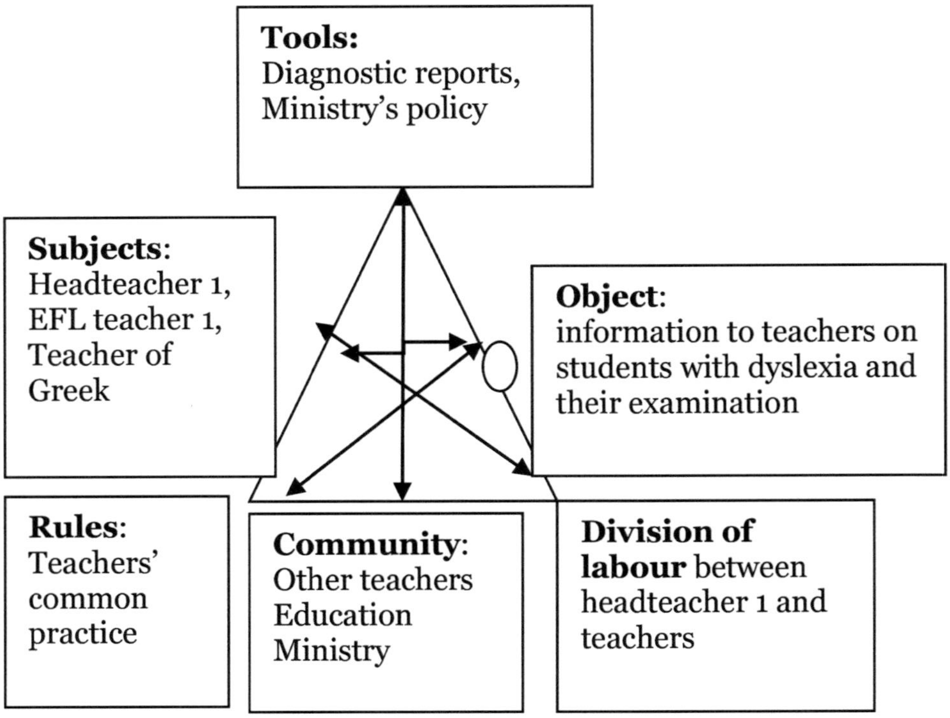

Figure 6.
Headteacher 1-EFL teacher 1 collaboration.

dyslexia and on how she can examine them. The headteacher's object is to inform teachers in his school about the students with dyslexia. However, it seems that the he did not inform teachers at the beginning of the year (September–October). Therefore, his object was not met by him but by the junior high school teacher who informed the EFL teacher about George's diagnosis. It is possible that headteacher 1 and EFL teacher 1 collaborated in the middle of the school year regarding the diagnostic reports since EFL teacher 1 seemed to know about them as I mentioned before.

In this section, I showed that in School 1 EFL teacher 1 and a teacher of Greek would have liked to be informed by the headteacher on the students with dyslexia but this did not happen in the beginning of the school year. EFL teacher 1 was informed by a teacher of Greek from the lower secondary school instead.

2.4 Collaboration between EFL teacher and teachers of Greek in School 1

Next, I discuss the collaboration between EFL teacher 1 and the teachers of Greek in School 1 around the examination of students with dyslexia.

EFL teacher 1 admitted that she does not collaborate with teachers of Greek of the same school as she believes that in Greek subjects the oral examination is much easier than in EFL even if the student with dyslexia is weak in the subject in which s/he is examined:

Extract 11. Interview with T1.

M And with the teachers of Greek? You said you haven't talked to them.
T1 I haven't talked to them because, look, they deal with Greek. The oral examination is much easier. How can I examine him orally in a foreign language? That is, it is as if I am asking someone who doesn't speak Greek to be examined orally in

> *Greek. In what can I examine him exactly? I talk to him let's say and he doesn't [talk back].*

The second generation of activity system is used for this theme as both EFL teacher 1 and the teacher of Greek belong to the same institution (School 1) and therefore the same community. The EFL teacher's object (object in **Figure 7**) was to have information on how they learn better and what difficulties they face and her goal was to examine the students with dyslexia like George orally (goal).

The teacher of Greek who taught George's class wanted to be informed on the students with dyslexia in her class (object) but this did not happen in the beginning of the school year (Extract 9). She was also interested in examining students orally (goal) when I told her that George wanted to be examined orally:

Extract 12. Field notes.

> *Therefore, there is a systemic contradiction in the activity system of School 1 (Figure 7) in the lack of an appropriate tool (how artifact) for the information of teachers on dyslexia issues and the establishment of collaboration among them.*

Therefore, there is a systemic contradiction in the activity system of School 1 (**Figure 7**) in the lack of an appropriate tool (how artifact) for the information of teachers on dyslexia issues and the establishment of collaboration among them.

2.5 Inter-collegial collaboration in School 2

Headteacher 2 told me that she informs teachers about dyslexia issues, on dyslexia diagnoses in the school and on the relevant guidelines:

Extract 13. Interview with HT2.

> *HT2 we give ... information to teachers around the problem and the dyslexia certificate as well as the relevant guidelines.*

It seems that headteacher 2 did inform the staff in her school about the above issues as EFL teacher 2 was fully informed about the students with dyslexia when

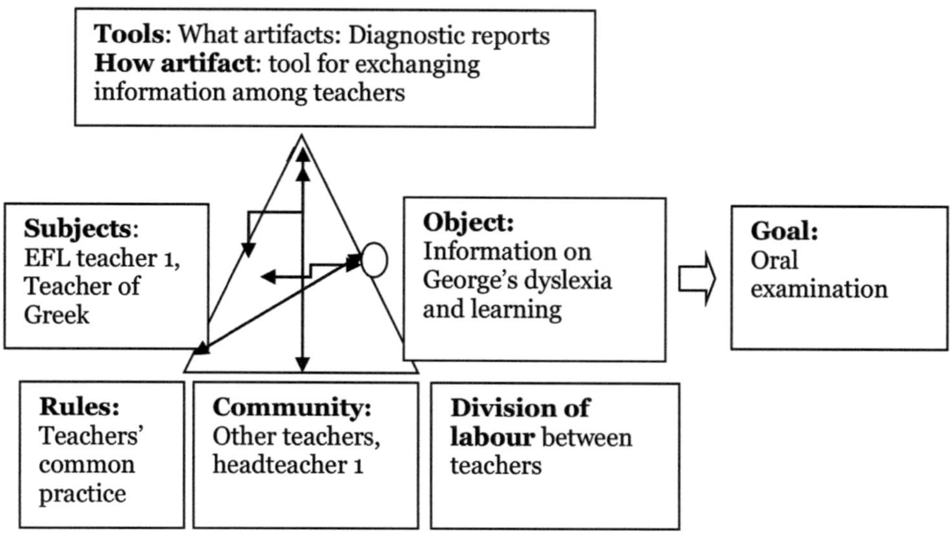

Figure 7.
Information on George's learning.

I first discussed the issue with her. EFL teacher 2 was also informed about the Education Ministry's guidelines regarding students with dyslexia. Therefore, headteacher 2's object of informing the teachers about students with dyslexia diagnoses and about the guidelines was achieved (**Figure 8**).

However, EFL teacher 2 was not aware of School 2's collaboration with the diagnostic centres that headteacher 2 told me about. This suggests that headteacher 2 has not informed EFL teacher 2 on the issue, which means that her object of informing teachers was partially met.

I also asked EFL teacher 2 if she collaborates with teachers of Greek in her school and she replied that when a teacher in the school suspects that a student has dyslexia s/he discusses it with the other teachers (Extract 14, lines 384–385). She asks what

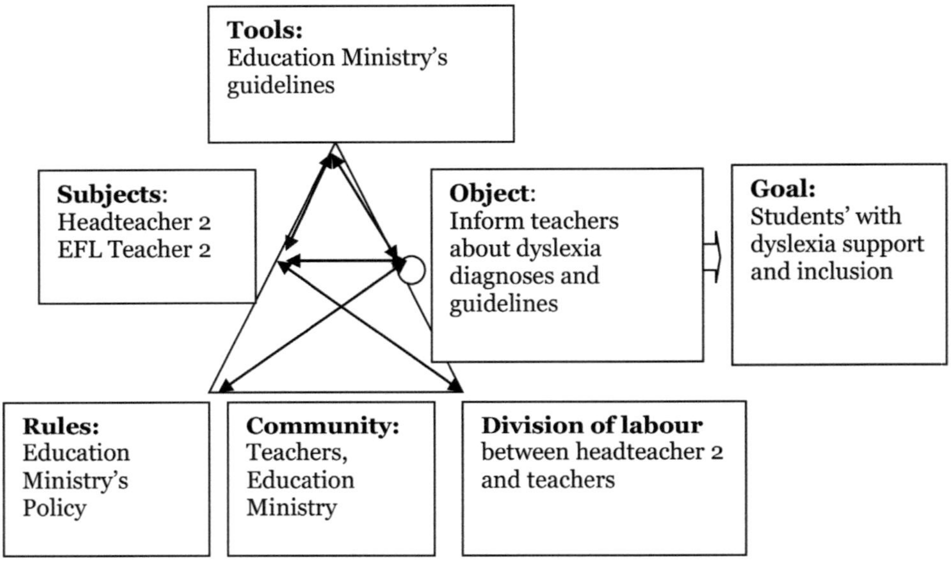

Figure 8.
Information from headteacher 2 to teachers.

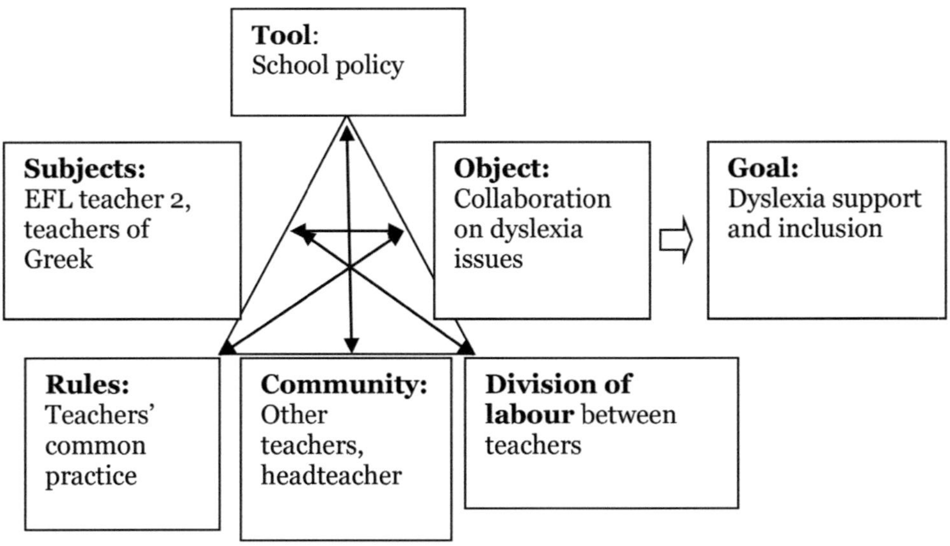

Figure 9.
Collaboration of EFL teacher 2 with teachers of Greek.

other teachers do in their classes only if she has a serious problem and if the student cannot follow the lesson at all (lines 389–391).

Extract 14. Interview with T2.

M Is there collaboration with teachers of Greek ... ?
T2 When someone suspects there is an issue s/he discusses it with the other colleagues to see if something is going on. If an issue arises, of course we discuss it
M To see what the others do, how the student behaves in their lesson and such.
T2 Only if I have a serious problem.
M Mmm.
T2 And I see that a child can't follow the lesson at all ...

In **Figure 9**, EFL teacher 2's and teachers' of Greek object of collaboration on dyslexia issues is met. Furthermore, in School 2, headteacher 2 effectively informs teachers about students' diagnoses and the guidelines from the Ministry of Education.

3. Conclusion

In this chapter, data related to the themes of collaboration across schools and inter-collegial collaboration were analysed. The analysis showed that the collaboration of colleagues in the same school was not effective in School 1, which influenced dyslexia provision offered by the EFL teachers and other teachers. On the other hand, collaboration of colleagues in the same school was more effective in School 2. Therefore, second generation of activity theory was used to the extent that the data allowed its use and it was demonstrated by the analysis that inter-organizational learning and boundary crossing did not take place in my study. This happened because my study is not an intervention study that aims to bring professionals from different backgrounds together to work on a common object.

This study demonstrated that a 'how artifact' is needed in order for the contradiction of the lack of communication between colleagues to be resolved. A staff meeting is necessary in secondary schools in the beginning of the school year in which headteachers inform teachers on the students' with dyslexia diagnoses. Regular staff meetings need to be organized during the school year in order for teachers of the same school to exchange information on students' with dyslexia difficulties, behavioural problems and progress and the teaching techniques they use. According to Mackay and Hunter-Carsch and Pollock and Waller, portraits or profiles on all pupils with specific learning difficulties need to be available to all staff in schools [1–3].

Acknowledgements

I would like to thank the teachers, the parents and the students who participated in this study and the University of Birmingham for funding this study.

Author details

Maria Rontou
Hellenic Open University, Loutraki, Greece

*Address all correspondence to: mariarontou720@hotmail.com

References

[1] Mackay N. The case for dyslexia-friendly schools. In: Reid G, Fawcett A, editors. Dyslexia in Context: Research, Policy and Practice. London: Whurr; 2004

[2] Hunter-Carsch M. Learning support in the secondary school: Needs analysis and provision for dyslexic students. In: Hunter-Carsch M, Herrington M, editors. Dyslexia and Effective Learning in Secondary and Tertiary Education. London: Whurr Publishers; 2001. pp. 12-37

[3] Pollock J, Waller E. Day-to-Day Dyslexia in the Classroom. London: Routledge; 1994

[4] Arapogianni A. Investigating the Approaches that Teachers in Greece Use to Meet the Needs of Children with Dyslexia in Secondary Schools. Birmingham: University of Birmingham; 2004

[5] Lappas N. Specific Learning Difficulties in Scotland and Greece: Perceptions and Provision [unpublished PhD thesis]. Stirling: University of Stirling; 1997

[6] Engestrom Y. Expansive learning at work: Toward an activity theoretical reconceptualization. Journal of Education and Work. 2001;**14**(1):133-156

[7] Vygotsky LS. Mind in Society: The Development of Higher Psychological Processes. Cambridge: Harvard University Press; 1978

[8] Vygotsky LS. Thought and Language. Cambridge, MA: MIT Press; 1987

[9] Martin D. A new paradigm to inform inter-professional learning for integrating speech and language provision into secondary schools: A socio-cultural activity theory approach. Child Language Teaching and Therapy. 2008;**24**(2):173-192

[10] Leont'ev AN. Activity, Consciousness, and Personality. Englewood Cliffs: Prentice-Hall; 1978

[11] Leont'ev AN. Problems of the Development of the Mind. Progress: Moscow; 1981

[12] Daniels H. Activity theory, discourse and Bernstein. Educational Review. 2004;**56**(2):121-132

[13] Davydov VV. The content and unsolved problems of activity theory. In: Engestrom Y, Miettinen R, Punamaki RL, editors. Perspectives on Activity Theory. Cambridge: Cambridge University Press; 1999. pp. 39-51

[14] Leadbetter J. The role of mediating artefacts in the work of educational psychologists during consultative conversations in schools. Educational Review. 2004;**56**(2):133-145

[15] Engestrom Y, Engestrom R, Vahaaho T. When the centre does not hold: The importance of knotworking. In: Chaiklin S, Hedegaard M, Jensen U, editors. Activity Theory and Social Practice. Aarhus: Aarhus University Press; 1999

[16] Engestrom Y. Innovative learning in work teams: Analysing cycles of knowledge creation in practice. In: Engestrom Y, Miettinen R, Punamaki RL, editors. Perspectives on Activity Theory. Cambridge: Cambridge University Press; 1999. pp. 377-404

[17] Denscombe M. The Good Research Guide for Small-Scale Social Research Projects. 2nd ed. Maidenhead: Open University Press; 2003

[18] Robson C. Real World Research: A Resource for Social Scientists and

Practitioner-Researchers. 2nd ed. Oxford: Blackwell; 2002

[19] Marshall C, Rossman GB. Designing Qualitative Research. London: Sage; 1995

[20] Brewer JD. Ethnography. Buckingham: Open University Press; 2000

[21] Cohen L, Manion L, Morrison M. Research Methods in Education. London: Routledge; 2007

[22] Fine GA, Shulman D. Lies from the field: Ethical issues in organizational ethnography. In: Ybema S, Yanow D, Wells H, Kamsteeg F, editors. Organizational Ethnography: Studying the Complexities of Everyday Life. London: Sage; 2009. pp. 177-195

[23] Delamont S. Fieldwork in Educational Settings: Methods, Pitfalls and Perspectives. London: Routledge; 2002

Chapter 11

The Child with Learning Difficulties and His Writing: A Study of Case

Edgardo Domitilo Gerardo Morales

Abstract

The purpose of this paper is to present one child with learning difficulties writing process in multigrade rural elementary school in México. It presents Alejandro's case. This boy lives in a rural area. He shows special educational needs about learning. He never had specialized attention because he lives in a marginalized rural area. He was integrated into regular school, but he faced some learning difficulties. He was always considered as a student who did not learn. He has coursed 2 years of preschool and 1 year of elementary school. Therefore, this text describes how child writes a list of words with and without image as support. Analysis consists to identify the child's conceptualizations about writing, his ways of approaching, and difficulties or mistakes he makes. The results show that Alejandro identifies letters and number by using pseudo-letters and conventional letter. These letters are in an unconventional position. There is no relationship grapheme and phoneme yet, and he uses different writing rules. We consider his mistakes as indicators of the learning process.

Keywords: writing difficulties, learning difficulties, writing learning, writing process, special education

1. Introduction

One of the purposes of Mexican education system is that students acquire conventional writing during first grades in elementary school [1]. This purpose consists of students to understand the alphabetical code, its meaning, and functionality. In this way, they can integrate into a discursive community.

The elementary school teacher teaches a heterogeneous group of children [1, 2]. Some students show different acquisition levels of the writing. This is due to literacy environment that the family and society provide. Thus, some children have had great opportunities to interact with reading and writing practices than others. Therefore, some students do not learn the alphabetical principle of writing at the end of the scholar year. They show characteristics of initial or intermediate acquisition level of the writing. In this way, it is difficult for children to acquire writing at the same time, at the term indicated by educational system or teachers.

In addition, there may be children with learning difficulties in the classroom. Department of Special Education teaches some children. Students with special educational needs show more difficulties to learn than their classmates [3].

They require more resources to achieve the educational objectives. These authors point out that special educational needs are relative. These needs arise between students' personal characteristics and their environment. Therefore, any child may have special educational needs, even if he/she does not have any physical disability. However, some students with learning difficulties do not have a complete assessment about their special educational needs. On the one hand, their school is far from urban areas; on the other hand, there are not enough teachers of special education for every school. In consequence, school teachers do not know their students' educational needs and teach in the same way. Thereby, students with learning difficulties do not have the necessary support in the classroom.

Learning difficulties of writing may be identified easily. Children with special educational needs do not learn the alphabetical principle of writing easily; that is, they do not relate phoneme with grapheme. Therefore, children show their conceptualizations about writing in different ways. Sometimes, teachers censor their students' written productions because they do not write in a conventional way. Children with special educational needs are stigmatized in the classroom. They are considered as less favored. At the end of the scholar year, children do not pass.

Therefore, the purpose of this paper is to present one child with special educational needs writing process in a Mexican multigrade rural school. This text describes how the child writes a list of words with and without image as support. Analysis consists to identify the child's conceptualizations about writing [4], his ways of approaching, and difficulties or mistakes he makes. These mistakes are the indicators of learning process [5].

This paper presents Alejandro's case. This boy lives in a rural area. He shows special educational needs about learning. He never had specialized attention because he lives in a marginalized rural area. He was integrated into regular school, but he faced some learning difficulties. He was always considered as a student who does not learn. Therefore, this text describes Alejandro's writing, what he does after 2 years of preschool and 1 year of elementary school.

2. Children with learning difficulties and their diagnosis

According to the National Institute for the Evaluation of Education [6], Mexican education system provides basic education (preschool, elementary, and secondary school) for students with special educational needs. There are two types of special attention: Center of Multiple Attention (CAM, in Spanish) and Units of Service and Support to Regular Education (USAER, in Spanish). In the first one, children with special educational needs go to this Center. These children receive attention according to basic education and their educational needs. In the second, specialized teachers on special education go to school and provide support to students. These teachers provide information to school teachers too. In this way, there is educational equity and inclusion in Mexican school [7].

Mexican education system proposes the psycho-pedagogical assessment to identifying students with special educational needs [3]. Teacher identifies student with more difficulties. Specialized teacher applies several predetermined tests individually. This assessment is organized as follows:

1. **Physical appearance**: Teacher describes the child's physical characteristics. These features indicate the type of food the student eats, care his or her person, the parents' attention, among other elements.

2. **Behavior observed during the assessment**: In this section, the teacher should record the conditions in which the assessment was carried out: child's attitude, behavior, and interest.

3. **Child's development history**: This section presents conditions in which pregnancy developed, physical development (ages in which child held his/her head, sat, crawled, walked, etc.), language development (verbal response to sounds and voices, age in which said his/her first words and phrases, etc.), family (characteristics of their family and social environment, frequent activities, etc.), hetero-family history (vision, hearing, etc.), medical history (health conditions, diseases, etc.), and scholar history (age at which he/she started school, type of school, difficulties, etc.).

4. **Present condition**: In this, there are four aspects:

    a. It refers to student's general aspects: intellectual area (information processing, attention, memory, understanding, etc.), motor development area (functional skills to move, take objects, position of his/her body, etc.), communicative-linguistic area (phonological, semantic, syntactic and pragmatic levels), adaptation and social interaction area (the child's skills to initiate or maintain relationships with others), and emotional area (the way of perceiving the world and people). In each one, it mentions the instruments he suggests, although there is not enough information about them [3].

    b. The second aspect is the curricular competence level. Teacher identifies what the student is capable of doing in relation to established purposes and contents by official curriculum.

    c. The third aspect is about the learning style and motivation to learn. It presents physical-environmental conditions where the child works, their interests, level attention, strategies to solve a task, and the incentives he receives.

    d. The fourth aspect is information about the student's environment: factors of the school, family, and social context that influence the child's learning.

Psycho-pedagogical assessment allows to identify children's general educational needs. In this way, the school teacher could have information about the students' difficulties. However, it is a general assessment. It contains several aspects and does not go deeper into one.

Therefore, this paper does not propose a new assessment. It consists of presenting one child's writing difficulties, his ways of conceptualizing writing, and some mistakes he gets to make.

3. Students with learning difficulties and their scholar integration

Since 1993, Mexican system education has tried to offer special education services to students with special educational needs in basic education [8]. The first step was to promote the integration of these children in regular education classrooms. However, only insertion of the student in the school was achieved. Therefore, the system of education searched for mechanisms to provide advice to teacher. In this way, student with learning difficulties can be attended at the same time in the classroom [8].

Educational integration has been directly associated with attention of students with learning difficulties, with or without physical disabilities [8]. However, this process implies a change in the school. For this, it is necessary to provide information and to create awareness to the educational community, permanent updating of teachers, joint work between teacher, family, and specialized teachers.

At present, Mexican education system looks at educational integration as process in which every student with learning difficulties is supported individually [9]. Adapting the curriculum to the child is the purpose of educational integration.

Curricular adequacy is one of the actions to support students with learning difficulties [10, 11]. This is an individualized curriculum proposal. Its purpose is to attend the students' special educational needs [3]. At present, Mexican education system indicates that there should be a curricular flexibility to promote learning processes. However, it is important to consider what the child knows about particular knowledge.

Regarding the subject of the acquisition of written language, it is necessary to know how the children build their knowledge about written. It is not possible to make a curricular adequacy if teachers do not have enough information about their students. However, children are considered as knowledge builders. Therefore, there are learning difficulties at the process.

4. Alejandro's case

This section presents Alejandro's personal information. We met him when we visited to his school for other research purposes. We focused on him because the boy was silent in class. He was always in a corner of the work table and did not do the activities. For this, we talked with his teacher and his mother to know more about him.

Alejandro is a student of an elementary multigrade rural school. He was 7 years old at the time of the study. He was in the second grade of the elementary school. His school is located in the region of the "Great Mountains" of the state of Veracruz, Mexico. It is a rural area, marginalized. To get to this town from the municipal head, it is necessary to take a rural taxi for half an hour. Then, you have to walk on a dirt road for approximately 50 min.

Alejandro's family is integrated by six people. He is the third of the four sons. He lives with his parents. His house is made of wood. His father works in the field: farming of corn, beans, and raising of sheep. His mother is a housewife and also works in the field. They have a low economic income. Therefore, they receive a scholarship. One of his older brothers also showed learning difficulties at school. His mother says both children have a learning problem. But, they do not have any money for attending their sons' learning difficulties. In addition, there are no special institutes near their house.

The boy has always shown learning difficulties. He went to preschool for 2 years. However, he did not develop the necessary skills at this level. At classes, this child was silent, without speaking. Preschool teachers believed that he was mute. Nevertheless, at scholar recess, he talked with his classmates. Alejandro was slow to communicate with words in the classroom.

When he started elementary school, Alejandro continued to show learning difficulties. At classes, he was silent too. He just watched what his classmates did. He did not do anything in the class. He took his notebook out of his backpack and just made some lines. Occasionally, he talked with his classmates. When the teacher asked him something, Alejandro did not answer. He looked down and did not answer. He just ducked his head and stayed for several minutes.

When Alejandro was in second grade, he did different activities than his classmates. His teacher drew some drawings for him and he painted these drawings. Other occasions, the teacher wrote some letters for him to paint. The child did every exercise during several hours. He did not finish his exercises quickly. Sometimes he painted some drawings during 2 h.

Although Alejandro requires specialized attention, he has not received it. He has not had a full psycho-pedagogical assessment at school by specialized teachers. His school does not have these teachers. Also, the child was not submitted to neurological structural examination or neurophysiological studies to exclude an organic origin of his learning difficulties. His parents do not have enough financial resources to do this type of study for him. In addition, one specialized institution that can do this type of study for free is in Mexico City. It is so far from child's house. It would be expensive for the child's parents. Therefore, he is only attended as a regular school student.

For this reason, this paper is interested in the boy's writing process. This is because Alejandro coursed 2 years of preschool and 1 year of elementary school; however, he does not show a conventional writing yet. In this way, it is interesting to analyze his conceptualizations about writing and difficulties he experiences.

5. Methodology

The purpose of this paper is to know the child's ways to approach writing spontaneously and his knowledge about the writing system. For this, the author used a clinical interview. He took into account the research interview guide "Analysis of Disturbances in the Learning Process of Reading and Writing" [12].

The clinical interview was conducted individually. We explored four points, but we only present two in this text: to write words and to write for image.

Interviewer took the child to the library room at school. There were no other students. First, the interviewer gave the child a sheet and asked to write his name. Alejandro wrote his name during long time. Interviewer only asked what it says there. He answered his name: "Alejandro." Next, the interviewer asked the child to write some letters and numbers he knew. Alejandro wrote them. The interviewer asked about every letter and number. The child answered "letter" or "number," and its name.

Next, the two writing tasks were the following:

1. *To write words*: The interviewer asked the child to write a group of words from the same semantic field in Spanish (because Alejandro is from Mexico) and one sentence. Order of words was from highest to lowest number of syllables. In this case, interviewer used semantic field of animals. Therefore, he used following words: GATO (cat), MARIPOSA (butterfly), CABALLO (horse), PERRO (dog), and PEZ (fish). The sentence was: EL GATO BEBE LECHE (The cat drinks milk). The interviewer questioned every written word. He asked the child to show with his finger how he says in every written production.

2. *To write for image*: This task was divided into two parts. The first analyzed the size and second analyzed the number.

Interviewer used the following image cards: horse-bird and giraffe-worm (**Figure 1**). Every pair of cards represents a large animal and a small animal.

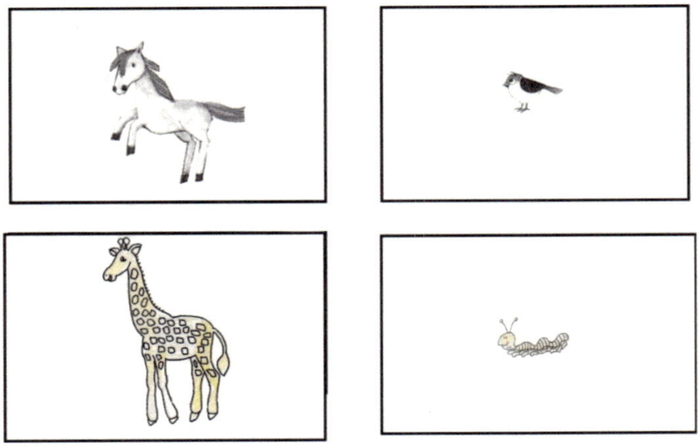

Figure 1.
Cards with large and small animals.

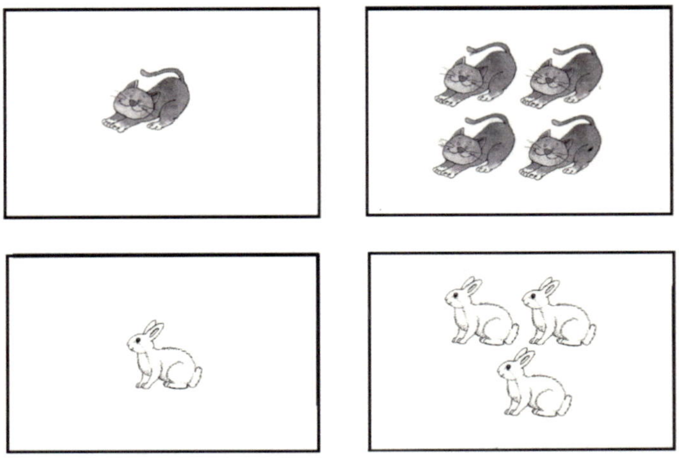

Figure 2.
Cards for singular and plural.

The purpose of this first task was to explore how the child writes when he looks at two images of animals with different size. The animal names have three syllables in Spanish: CA-BA-LLO (horse), PA-JA-RO (bird), etc. In this way, we can see how the child writes.

The interviewer used the following pair of cards for second task (**Figure 2**).

First card shows one animal (singular) and the second shows some animals (plural). In this way, we search to explore how the child produces his writings when he observes one or more objects, if there are similarities or differences to write.

The interviewer asked what was in every card. Next, he asked the child to write something. Alejandro wrote something in every picture. Afterward, the interviewer asked the child to read every word that he wrote. Child pointed with his finger what he wrote.

After, the interview was transcribed for analysis. We read the transcription. The author analyzed every written production. He identified the child's conceptualizations about writing. He compared the written production and what the child said. In this way, the analysis did not only consist to identify the level of writing development. This text describes the child's writing, the ways in which he conceptualizes the writing, the difficulties he experienced to write, and his interpretations about writing.

6. Alejandro's writing

This section describes Alejandro's writing process. As we already mentioned, Alejandro is 7 years old and he studies in the second grade of the elementary school. His teacher says the child should have a conventional writing, because he has already coursed 1 year of elementary school, but it is not like that. Most of his classmates write a conventional way, but he does not.

We organized this section in three parts. The first part presents how Alejandro wrote his name and how he identifies letters and numbers; the second part refers to the writing of words; and the third part is writing for picture.

6.1 Alejandro writes his name and some letters and numbers

The first part of the task consisted of Alejandro writing his name and some letters and numbers he knows. His name was requested for two reasons. The first reason is to identify the sheet, because the interviewer interviewed other children in the same school. Also, it was necessary to identify every written productions of the group of students. The second reason was to observe the way he wrote his name and how he identified letters and numbers.

The interviewer asked the child to write his name at the top of the sheet. When the interviewer said the instructions, Alejandro was thoughtful during a long time. He was not pressed or interrupted. He did not do anything for several seconds. The child looked at the sheet and looked at everywhere. After time, he took the pencil and wrote the following on the sheet (**Figure 3**).

The interviewer looked at Alejandro's writing. He asked if something was lacking. The interviewer was sure that Alejandro knew his name and his writing was not complete. However, Alejandro was thoughtful, and looked at the sheet for a long time. The interviewer asked if his name was already complete. The child answered "no." The interviewer asked the child if he remembered his name. Alejandro denied with his head. So, they continued with another task.

Alejandro has built the notion of his name. We believe that he has had some opportunities to write his name. Perhaps, his teacher has asked him to write his name on his notebooks, as part of scholar work in the classroom. We observed that Alejandro used letters with conventional sound value. This is because he wrote three initial letters of his name: ALJ (Alejandro). The first two letters correspond to the beginning of his name. Then, he omits "E" (ALE-), and writes "J" (ALJ). However, Alejandro mentions that he does not remember the others. This may show that he has memorized his name, but at that moment he failed to remember the others, or, these letters are what he remembers.

Subsequently, the interviewer asked Alejandro to write some letters and numbers he knew. The sequence was: a letter, a number, a letter, another letter, and number. In every Alejandro' writing, the interviewer asked the child what he wrote. In this way, Alejandro wrote the following (**Figure 4**).

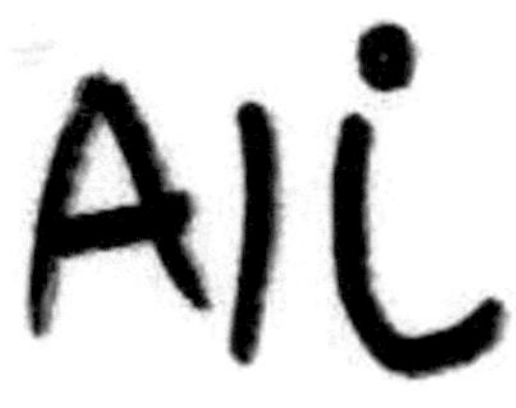

Figure 3.
Alejandro's name.

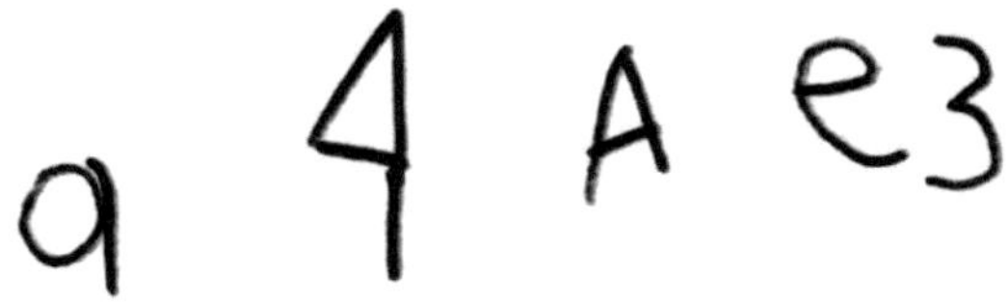

Figure 4.
Letters and numbers written by Alejandro.

For this task, Alejandro wrote for a long time. He did not hurry to write. He looked at sheet and wrote. The child looked at the interviewer, looked at the sheet again and after a few seconds he wrote. The interviewer asked about every letter or number.

We can observe that Alejandro differentiates between letter and number. He wrote correctly in every indication. That is, when the interviewer asked him to write a letter or number, he did so, respectively. In this way, Alejandro knows what he needs to write a word and what is not, what is for reading and what is not.

Also, we can observe that the child shows a limited repertoire of letters. He did not write consonants. He used only vowels: A (capital and lower) and E (lower). It shows us that he differentiates between capital and lower letter. Also, he identifies what vowels and letters are because the child answered which they were when the interviewer asked about them.

6.2 Writing words from the same semantic field

Asking the child to write words spontaneously is a way to know what he knows or has built about the writing system [12]. Although we know Alejandro presents learning difficulties and has not consolidated a conventional writing, it is necessary to ask him to write some words. This is for observing and analyzing what he is capable of writing, what knowledge he has built, as well as the difficulties he experiences.

The next picture presents what Alejandro wrote (**Figure 5**). We wrote the conventional form in Spanish next to every word. We wrote these words in English in the parentheses too.

At the beginning of the interview, Alejandro did not want to do the task. He was silent for several seconds. He did not write anything. He looked at the sheet and the window. The interviewer insisted several times and suspended the recording to encourage the child to write. Alejandro mentioned he could not write, because he did not know the letters and so he would not do it. However, the interviewer insisted him. After several minutes, Alejandro took the pencil and started to write.

Alejandro wrote every word for 1 or 2 min. He required more seconds or minutes sometimes. He looked at the sheet and his around. He was in silence and looking at the sheet other times. We identified that he needs time to write. This shows that he feels insecure and does not know something for writing. He feels insecure because he was afraid of being wrong and that he was punished by the interviewer for it. It may be that in class he is penalized when he makes a mistake. There is ignorance because he does not know some letters, and he has a low repertoire of the writing system. Thus, Alejandro needs to think about writing and look for representing it. Therefore, this is why the child needs more time to write.

We identified that the child does not establish a phoneme-grapheme relationship. He only shows with his finger from left to right when he read every word. He does not establish a relationship with the letters he used. In each word, there is no correspondence with the number of letters. The child also does not establish a constant because there is variation in number and variety of letters sometimes.

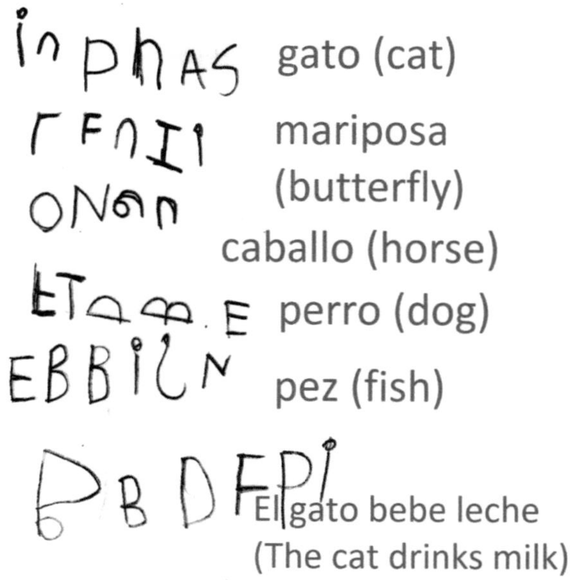

Figure 5.
List of words written by Alejandro.

Alejandro used letters unrelated to the conventional writing of the words. For example, when he wrote GATO (cat), Alejandro used the following letters: inpnAS. It is possible to identify that no letter corresponds to the word. Perhaps, Alejandro wrote those letters because they are recognized or remembered by him.

Alejandro shows a limited repertoire of conventional letters. This is observed when he uses four vowels: A, E, I, O. The child used these vowels less frequently. There is one vowel in every word at least. When Alejandro wrote PEZ (fish), he used two vowels. We observed that he writes these vowels at the beginning or end of the word. However, we do not know why he places them that way. Maybe this is a differentiating principle by him.

There is qualitative and quantitative differentiation in Alejandro's writing. That is, he did not write any words in the same way. All the words written by him are different. Every word has different number and variety of letters. When two words contain the same number of letter, they contain different letters.

When Alejandro wrote MARIPOSA (butterfly), he used five letters. The number of letters is less than what he used for GATO (cat). Maybe he wrote that because the interviewer said "butterfly is a small animal." This is because the cat is bigger than the butterfly. Therefore, it may be possible that he used lesser letters for butterfly.

In Spanish, PERRO (dog) contains five letters. Alejandro wrote five letters. In this case, Alejandro's writing corresponds to the necessary number of letters. However, it seems that there is no writing rules for him. This is for two reasons: first, because there is no correspondence with the animal size. Horse is larger than dog and Alejandro required lesser letters for horse than for dog. Second, CABALLO (horse) is composed by three syllables and PERRO (dog) by two. Alejandro used more letters to represent two syllables. In addition, it is observed that there is a pseudo-letter. It looks like an inverted F, as well as D and B, horizontally.

When Alejandro wrote PEZ (fish), the interviewer first asked how many letters he needed to write that word. The child did not answer. Interviewer asked for this again and student said that he did not know. Then, interviewer said to write PEZ (fish). For several minutes, Alejandro just looked the sheet and did not say anything. The interviewer questioned several times, but he did not answer. After several minutes, Alejandro wrote: E. The interviewer asked the child if he has finished. He denied with his head. After 1 min, he started to write. We observed that his writing contains six letters. Capital letters are predominated.

Alejandro used inverted letters in three words. They may be considered as pseudo-letters. However, if we observe carefully they are similar to conventional letters. The child has written them in different positions: inverted.

May be there is a writing rule by Alejandro. His words have a minimum of four letters and a maximum of six letters. This rule has been established by him. There is no relation to the length of orality or the object it represents.

We can identify that Alejandro shows a primitive writing [4]. He is still in writing system learning process. The phoneticization process is not present yet. The child has not achieved this level yet. He only uses letters without a conventional sound value. There is no correspondence to phoneme-grapheme, and he uses pseudo-letters sometimes.

6.3 To write for image

Write for image allows us to know what happens when the child writes something in front of an image [12]. It is identified if there is the same rules used by the child, number of letters, or if there is any change when he writes a new word. It may happen that the length of the words is related to the size of the image or the number of objects presented. In this way, we can identify the child's knowledge and difficulties when he writes some words.

6.3.1 The image size variable

The first task is about observing how the child writes when he is in front of two different sized images. That is, we want to identify if the image size influences on his writings. Therefore, two pairs of cards were presented to Alejandro. Every pair of cards contained two animals, one small and one large. The interviewer asked Alejandro to write the name on each one (**Figure 6**).

Based on the writing produced by Alejandro, we mentioned the following:

Alejandro delimits his space to write. When he wrote for first pair of words, the child drew a wide rectangle and he made an oval and several squares for the second pair of words. The child wrote some letters to fill those drawn spaces. It seems that Alejandro's rule is to fill the space and not only represent the word.

When Alejandro writes the words, we identified that he presents difficulty in the conventional directionality of writing. He wrote most of words from left to right (conventional directionality), but he wrote some words from right to left (no conventional). For example, the child started to write the second word on the left.

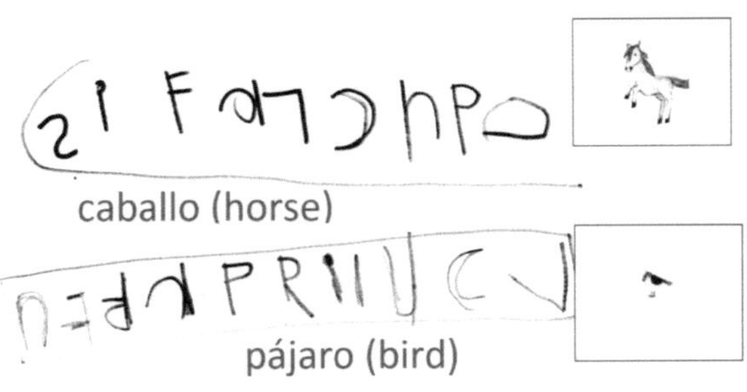

Figure 6.
Horse and bird writing.

He wrote seven letters. He looked at the sheet for some seconds. After, he continued to write other letters on the right. He wrote and completed the space he had left, from right to left.

Alejandro shows two ways to write: left–right (conventional) and right–left (no conventional). When he wrote the last word, the child wrote one letter under another. There was no limited space on the sheet. Alejandro wrote it there. The child has not learned the writing directionality.

When we compared Alejandro's writings, we identified that the number of letters used by him does not correspond to the image size. Although the images were present and he looked them when he wrote, the child took into account other rules to write. The six names of animals had three syllables in Spanish and Alejandro used nine letters for CABALLO (horse) and eleven for PÁJARO (bird). The letters used by him are similar to the conventional ones. However, these are in different positions. There are no phonetic correspondences with the words. The child shows a primitive writing. Alejandro has not started the level of relation between phoneme and grapheme yet. We can believe that the boy wrote some letters to cover the space on the sheet. Alejandro takes into account the card size instead of the image size.

After writing a list of words, the interviewer asked Alejandro to read and point out every word he wrote. The purpose of this task is to observe how the child relates his writing to the sound length of the word. When Alejandro read CABALLO (horse), he pointed out as follows (**Figure 7**).

Alejandro reads every word and points out what he reads. In this way, he justifies what he has written. In the previous example, Alejandro reads the first syllable and points out the first letter, second syllable with the second letter. At this moment, he gets in conflict when he tries to read the third syllable. It would correspond to the third letter. However, "there are more letters than he needs." When he reads the word, he shows the beginning of phoneticization: relation between one syllable with one letter. This is the syllabic writing principle [4]. Nevertheless, he has written more letters. Therefore, Alejandro says "o" in the other letters. In this way, we can point out that Alejandro justifies every letters and there is a correspondence between what he reads and what he writes.

When Alejandro reads the second word, the child pointed out as follows (**Figure 8**).

Alejandro makes a different correspondence syllable-letter than the first word. Although his writing was in two ways, his reading is only one direction: from left to right. The first syllable is related to first three letters he wrote. The second syllable is related to the fourth letter. But, he faces the same problem as in the previous word: "there are many letters." So he justifies the other letters as follows. He reads the third syllable in relation to the sixth and seventh letter. And, reads "o" for the other letters.

When interviewer showed the next pair of cards, Alejandro wrote as following (**Figure 9**).

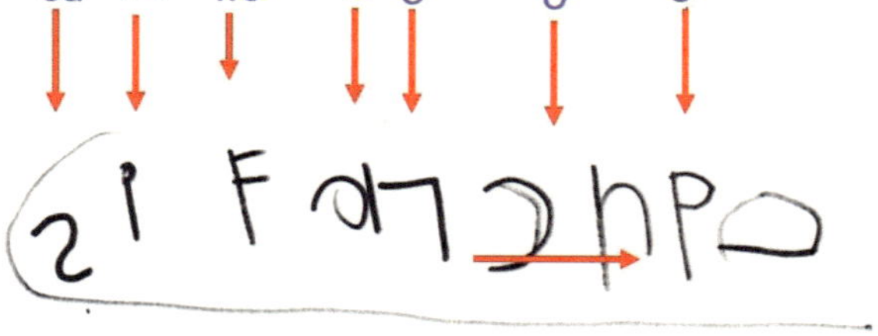

Figure 7.
Alejandro reads "caballo" (horse).

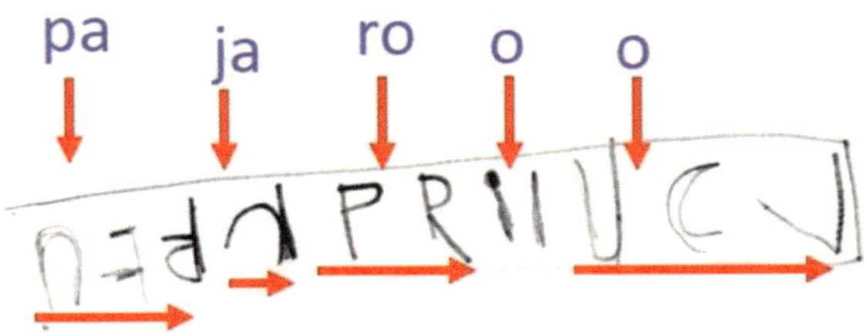

Figure 8.
Alejandro reads "pájaro" (bird).

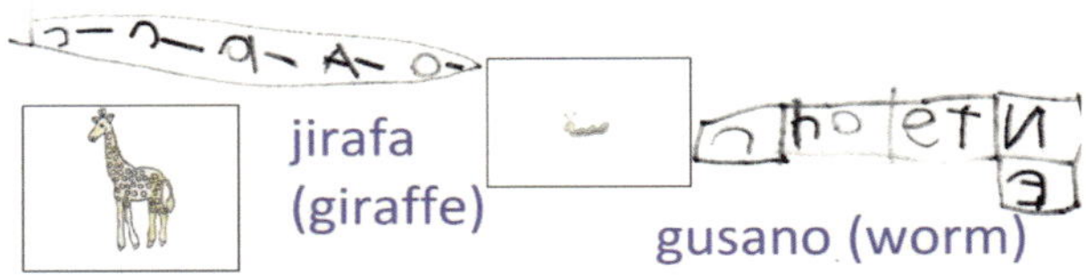

Figure 9.
Giraffe and worm writing by Alejandro.

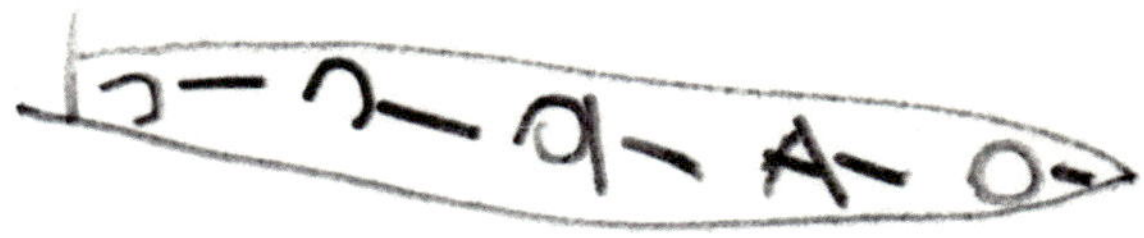

Figure 10.
Giraffe writing.

When the interviewer shows the pair of cards to Alejandro, the child said "It's a zebra." So, the interviewer said "It's a giraffe and it's a worm" and pointed out every card. The interviewer asked Alejandro to write the name of every animal. First, the child draws a rectangle across the width of the sheet. Next, he started to write on the left side inside the rectangle. He said the first syllable "JI" while writing the first letter. After, he said "ra," he wrote a hyphen. Then, he said "e" and wrote another letter. At that moment, he looked at the sheet and filled the space he left with some letters (**Figure 10**).

Alejandro shows different rules of writing. These rules are not the same as previous. He delimited the space to write and filled the space with some letters. The child tries to relate the syllable with one letter, but he writes others. There is a limited repertoire of letters too. In this case, it seems that he used the same letters: C capital and lower letter, A capital and lower letter, and O. We believe that he uses hyphens to separate every letter. However, when he wrote the first hyphen, it reads the second syllable. We do not know why he reads there. Alejandro had tried to use conventional letters. He uses signs without sound value. In addition, there is no relation phoneme and grapheme.

When Alejandro wrote GUSANO (worm), he drew a rectangle and divided it into three small squares. Then, he drew other squares below the previous ones. After, he began to write some letters inside the squares, as seen in the following picture (**Figure 11**).

Alejandro used other rules to write. They are different than the previous. Alejandro has written one or two letters into every box. At the end, he writes some letters under the last box. There is no correspondence between what he reads and writes. There are also no fixed rules of writing for him. Rather, it is intuited that he draws the boxes to delimit his space to write.

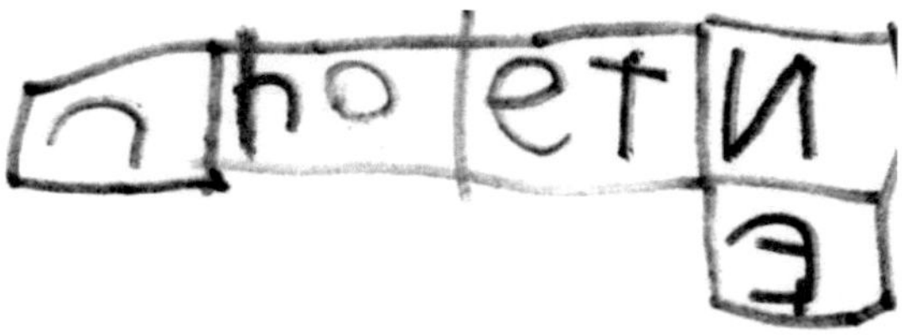

Figure 11.
Worm writing.

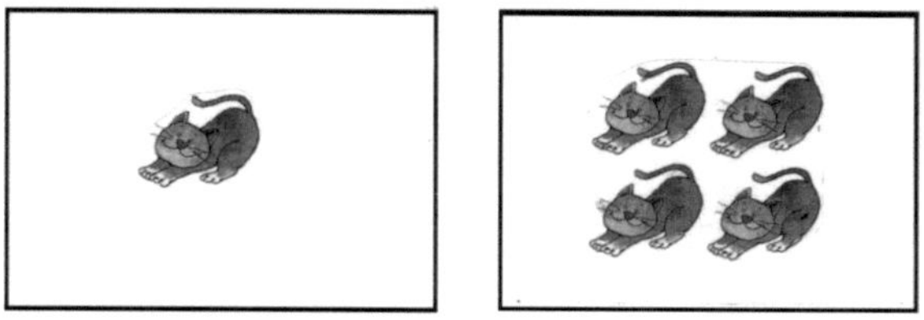

Figure 12.
Cards with one cat and four cats.

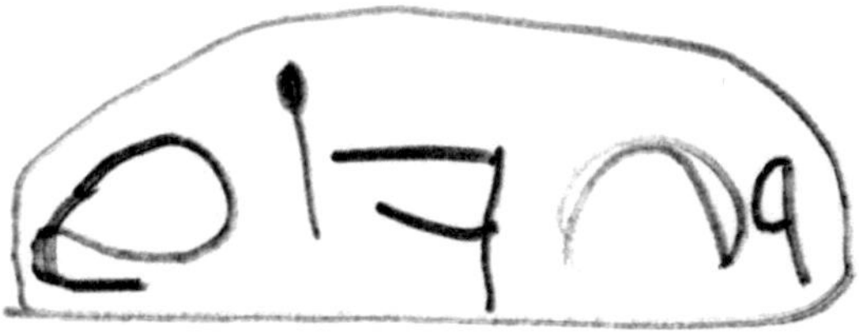

Figure 13.
Alejandro writes GATO (cat).

6.3.2 Singular and plural writing

The next task consists to write singular and plural. For this, the interviewer showed Alejandro the following images (**Figure 12**).

Alejandro drew an oval for first card. This oval is on the left half of the sheet. He wrote the following (**Figure 13**).

Next, the interviewer asked Alejandro to write for the second card, in plural. For this, Alejandro draws another oval from the middle of the sheet, on the right side. The child did not do anything for 1 h 30 min. After this time, he wrote some different letters inside the oval (**Figure 14**). He wrote from right to left (unconventional direction).

Alejandro wrote in the opposite conventional direction: from right to left. He tried to cover the delimited space by him. His letters are similar to the conventional ones. Also, there are differences between the first and the second word. He used lesser letters for first word than the second. That is, there are lesser letters for singular and more letters for plural. Perhaps, the child took into account the number of objects in the card.

The writing directionality may have been influenced by the image of the animals: cats look at the left side. Alejandro could have thought he was going to write from right to left, as well as images of the cards. Therefore, it is necessary to research how he writes when objects look at the right side. In this way, we can know if this influences the directionality of Alejandro's writing.

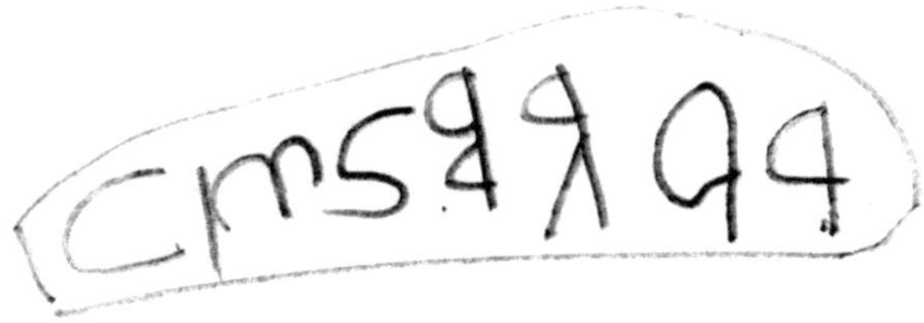

Figure 14.
Alejandro writes GATOS (cats).

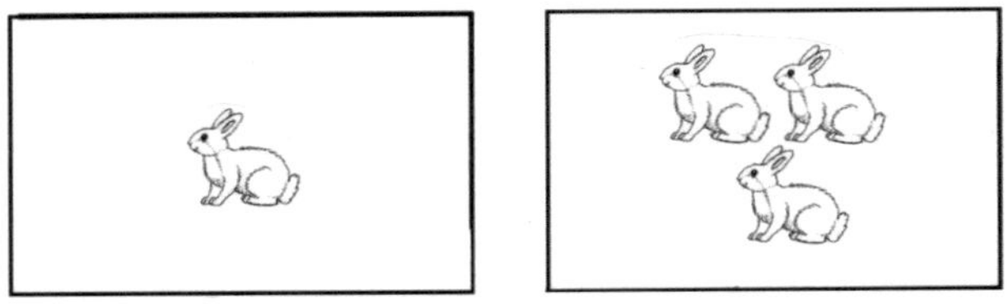

Figure 15.
Cards with one rabbit and three rabbits.

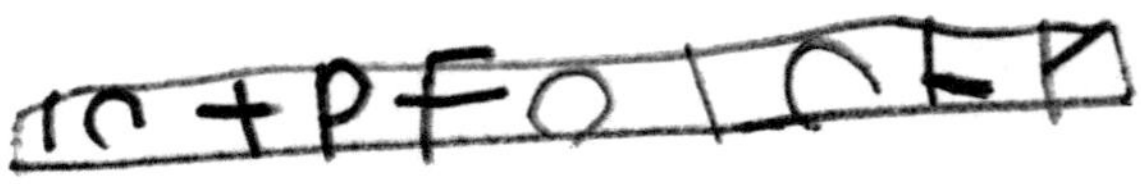

Figure 16.
Alejandro writes CONEJO (rabbit).

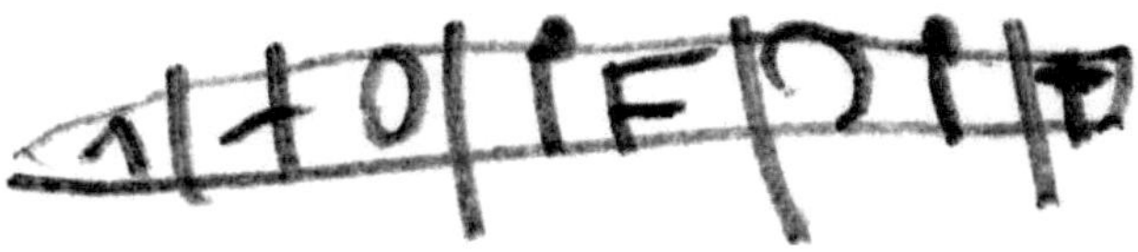

Figure 17.
Alejandro writes CONEJOS (rabbits).

With the next pair of images (**Figure 15**), the interviewer asked Alejandro to write CONEJO (rabbit) and CONEJOS (rabbits).

Alejandro draws a rectangle in the middle of the sheet for the first card (rabbit). He said "cone" (rab-) and wrote the first letter on the left of the sheet. Then, he said "jo" (bit) and wrote the second letter. He said "jo" again and wrote the third letter. He was thoughtful for some seconds. He started to write other letters. His writing is as follows (**Figure 16**).

At the beginning, Alejandro tries to relate the syllables of the word with first two letters. However, he justifies the other letters when he read the word. There is no exact correspondence between the syllable and the letter. As well as his writing is to fill the space he delimited.

Alejandro takes into account other rules for plural writing. He drew a rectangle across the width of the sheet. Starting on the left, he said "CO" and wrote one letter. Then, he said "NE" and drew a vertical line. After, he said "JO" and wrote other letters. His writing is as follows (**Figure 17**).

Alejandro writes both words differently. He reads CONEJO (rabbit) for first word and CONEJOS (rabbits) for the second. Both words are different from each other. But, he wrote them with different rules. This is confusing for us because there are vertical lines between every two letters in the second word. We believe that the child tried to represent every object, although he did not explain it.

In summary, Alejandro shows different writings. He used pseudo-letters and conventional letter. These letters are in unconventional positions. There is no relationship between grapheme and phoneme yet; and, he uses different writing rules.

7. Conclusions

We described Alejandro's writing process. According to this description, we can note the following:

Alejandro is a student of an elementary regular school. He presents learning difficulties. He could not write "correctly." However, he did not have a full assessment by specialized teachers. His school is so far from urban areas and his parents could not take him to a special institution. Therefore, he has not received special support. Also, there is not a favorable literacy environment in his home. His teacher teaches him like his classmates. Usually, he has been marginalized and stigmatized because "he does not know or work in class."

We focused on Alejandro because he was a child who was always distracted in class. We did not want to show his writing mistakes as negative aspects, but as part of his learning process. Errors are indicators of a process [5]. They inform the person's skills. They allow to identify the knowledge that is being used [13]. In this way, errors can be considered as elements with a didactic value.

Alejandro showed some knowledge and also some difficulties to write. The child identifies and distinguishes letters and numbers. We do not know if he conceptualizes their use in every one. When he wrote, he shows his knowledge: letters are for reading, because he did not use any number in the words.

The writing directionality is a difficulty for Alejandro. He writes from left to right and also from right to left. We do not know why he did that. We did not research his reasons. But, it is important to know if there are any factors that influence the child to write like this.

The student does not establish a phoneme-grapheme relationship yet. He is still in an initial level to writing acquisition. He uses conventional letters and pseudo-letters to write. There are no fixed rules to write: number and variety of letters. However, we observed student's thought about writing. He justifies his writings when he reads them and invents letters to represent some words.

There is still a limited repertoire of letters. He used a few letters of the alphabet. Therefore, Alejandro needs to interact with different texts, rather than teaching him letter by letter. Even if "he does not know those letters." In this way, he is going to appropriate other elements and resources of the writing system.

Time he takes to write is an important element for us. He refused to write for several minutes at the beginning. After, he wrote during 1 or 2 min every word. As we mentioned previously, we believe that Alejandro did not feel sure to do the task. Perhaps, he thought that the interviewer is going to penalize for his writing "incorrectly." He felt unable to write. Therefore, it is important that children's mistakes are not censored in the classroom. Mistakes let us to know the child's knowledge and their learning needs.

We considered that class work was not favorable for Alejandro. He painted letters, drawings, among others. These were to keep him busy. Therefore, it is important for the child to participate in reading and writing practices. In this way, he can be integrated into the scholar activities and is not segregated by his classmates.

About children with learning difficulties, it is important that these children write as they believe. Do not censor their writings. They are not considered as people incapable. It is necessary to consider that learning is a slow process. Those children will require more time than their classmates.

Special education plays an important role in Mexico. However, rather than attending to the student with learning difficulties in isolation, it is necessary that the teacher should be provided with information and the presence of specialized teachers in the classroom. In this way, the student with learning difficulties can be integrated into class, scholar activities, and reading and writing practices.

We presented Alejandro's writing process in this paper. Although he was considered as a child with learning difficulties, we identified he shows some difficulties, but he knows some elements of the writing system too.

Acknowledgements

I thank Alejandro, his parents, and his teacher for the information they provided to me about him.

Conflict of interest

The authors declare no conflict of interest.

Author details

Edgardo Domitilo Gerardo Morales
Faculty of Philosophy and Letters, National Autonomous University of Mexico, México City, México

*Address all correspondence to: edogemo@gmail.com

References

[1] SEP. Aprendizajes Clave Para la Educación Integral. Plan y Programas de Estudio Para la Educación Básica. México, D.F.: Secretaria de Educación Pública; 2017. ISBN: 970-57-0000-1

[2] SEP. Propuesta Educativa Multigrado 2005. México: Secretaria de Educación Pública; 2005

[3] García-Cedillo E, Escalante I, Escandón M, Fernández L, Mustre A, Puga I. La Integración Educativa en el Aula Regular. Principios, Finalidades y Estrategias. México: Secretaría de Educación Pública; 2000. ISBN: 978-607-8279-18-0

[4] Ferreiro E, Teberosky A. Los Sistemas de Escritura en el Desarrollo del Niño. México, D.F.: Editorial Siglo XXI; 1979. ISBN 968-23-1578-6

[5] Dolz J, Gagnon R, Vuillet Y. Production écrite et Difficultés D'apprentisage. Genève: Carnets des Sciences de L'education. Université de Genéve; 2011. ISBN: 2-940195-44-7

[6] INEE. Panorama Educativo de México. Indicadores del Sistema Educativo Nacional 2017. Educación Básica y Media Superior. México: Instituto Nacional para la Evaluación de la Educación; 2018

[7] SEP. Modelo Educativo: Equidad e Inclusión. México: Secretaria de Educación Pública; 2017. ISBN: 978-607-97644-4-9

[8] SEP. Orientaciones Generales Para el Funcionamiento de los Servicios de Educación Especial. México: Secretaria de Educación Pública; 2016. ISBN: 970-57-0016-8

[9] SEP. Estrategia de Equidad e Inclusión en la Educación Básica: Para Alumnos con Discapacidad, Aptitudes Sobresalientes y Dificultades Severas de Aprendizaje, Conducta o Comunicación. México, DF: Secretaria de Educación Pública; 2018

[10] Durán M. Las Adecuaciones Curriculares Individuales: Hacia la Equidad en Educación Especial. México: Secretaría de Educación Pública; 2016. ISBN 968-9082-33-7

[11] CONAFE. Discapacidad Intelectual. Guía Didáctica Para la Inclusión en Educación Inicial y Básica. México: Secretaria de Educación Pública; 2010

[12] Ferreiro E, Gómez M. Análisis de las Perturbaciones en el Proceso de Aprendizaje de la Lecto-Escritura. Fascículo 1. México: SEP-DGEE; 1982

[13] Vaca J. Así Leen (Textos) los Niños. Textos Universitarios. México: Universidad Veracruzana; 2006. ISBN: 968-834-753-1

Section 5

Strategy of Interventions in Learning Disabilities

Chapter 12

Transition Possibilities for Adolescents with Intellectual Disabilities into Adulthood

Rakgadi Grace Malapela and Gloria Thupayagale-Tshweneagae

Abstract

Transition possibilities for adolescents with intellectual disabilities into adulthood remain a complex issue and often neglected by the healthcare system and non-healthcare system. Given the responsibilities and roles that the healthcare system, non-healthcare system and families have to fulfil to address the transition possibility issue, the lack of knowledge, skills and resources negatively impacts on the transition possibility. In favour of situating adolescents with intellectual disabilities into adulthood, the provision and development of working skills need to be prioritised. Transition possibilities are to be considered to all adolescents with intellectual disabilities.

Keywords: adolescents, adulthood, intellectual disabilities, transition and possibility

1. Introduction

Adolescence is a time of transition, involving multidimensional changes, namely biological, psychological and social [1]. These changes occur simultaneously and at different paces for each adolescent. Extant literature reports that the world is home to 1.2 billion adolescents aged between 10 and 19 years. Transition for adolescents is not only biological, but it also includes emotional transition [2]. The United Nations statistics has reported that there are more than 600 million people with disability and that 80 million live in Africa. There is also an estimation that more than 300,000 adolescents have intellectual disabilities. Majority of adolescents with intellectual disabilities (IDs) adolescents would be excluded from acquiring some education and employment opportunities, as well as to suffer discrimination Nyangweso [3]. In addition, Meleis, Sawyer, Im, Messias, Schumacher [4] transition is perceived to be complicated. Adolescents with IDs will grow into adulthood as a result of improved healthcare and related technologies. Pandey and Agarwal [5] wrote that even though transitions are almost normal as they happen often, it is, however, very challenging for adolescents moving into adulthood especially for those with intellectual disabilities who may remain wholly dependent on their parents for emotional wellbeing.

This chapter provides a clear and detailed definition of the concept of transition, transition of adolescents with intellectual disabilities (IDs), followed by governmental intervention. Transition possibilities for adolescents with ID are discussed under various roles of the government, healthcare workers and communities.

2. Transition as a concept

The concept of 'transition' has been in existence for more than three decades. It is among the concepts that are debated on its meaning and uses in literature. Transitions occur throughout life and are the processes faced by all humans, from birth, to adolescence and to adulthood, from being immature to mature and from being dependent to independent [6]. Transition is often associated with movement from a more shielded environment to a more self-directed environment. It is characterised by the ability to make decisions and to take care of oneself [7]. Transition also includes many adjustments that have to occur in life. Such events include leaving parents to boarding school, leaving home after parental death to an orphanage and all other life events that may render one to transit from one area to another [8]. Chick and Meleis [9] summarises transition by defining it as 'a passage or movement from one state, condition or place to another' (p239). Ally et al. [10] are of the opinion that transitions are aimed at improving one's quality of life. It is a movement from one area of dependency to one area of independence, where one can do activities of daily living with minimal assistance. The authors further noted that it is about the cognitive and adaptive functioning of the individual. The process of transitioning is very difficult for most adolescents and could be particularly difficult for those adolescents with intellectual disabilities [11]. Shaw and DeLaet [12] define transition as a process, a point in time and a perception. As a process, transition needs people with ID their families, caregivers and the healthcare system to work together towards a common goal. The authors argue that transition entails the period starting from the anticipation of transition until the new status and change have been achieved. Lastly, the authors are of the view that transition depends on the individuals' interpretations of what transition mean to them rather than being an event. Furthermore, this depends upon the setting in which the transition process takes place. Eighteen years is globally believed to be an age of maturity, and hence adolescents when they turn 18 are expected to have reached a certain level of independence and are able to make life decisions such as employment and career. In accordance with Patterson and Pegg [13] past history reflects that adolescents with IDs were devalued and not allowed to live independently. These assumptions and beliefs pose challenges for those who are intellectually disabled.

3. Transition of adolescents with intellectual disabilities

Intellectual disability is characterised by several limitations in mental, emotional, cognitive and physical functioning. People with intellectual disabilities display very problematic behaviours that require attention at all times [14]. The definition of intellectual disability is also wrought with many controversies. To date there is no single definition that is acceptable for all. For instance, it is believed that people with intellectual disability's social and practical skills differ significantly from what is accepted as normal by his or her society (American Association of Intellectual and Developmental Disabilities (2011 cited in Aldersey [15])). On the contrary, Werner [16] and Lancaster et al. [17] define ID as characterised by significant limitations in intellectual functioning with an IQ below 75 which originates before the age of 18 years. To this end, intellectual disability has been defined by limitations in intellectual functioning and adaptive behaviours. They need more attention and assistance to cope with activities of daily living Shogren and Plotner [18].

The transition of adolescents with ID into adulthood is challenging in that they are expected to go through psychological and social maturation just like their able counterparts. There is a range of issues associated with transition of adolescents with ID into adulthood. They include rehabilitation and special education issues.

However, in most countries, especially developing countries, they do not have structures in place to assist them achieve this milestone [8]. Most often, there are no programmes and policies suited for addressing their needs.

Disability is a developing concept in Africa as it is entrenched within the culture [19]. In the African context, disability is associated with supernatural causes that affect the way family members would treat the individual with ID [20]. Aldersey [15] posits that disability in Africa is a formation of one's culture. Etiyiebo and Omiegbe [20] also support this view that culture defines an individual with intellectual disability as less than human. The two studies quoted above gave examples of other studies in Africa, such as Botswana, Zimbabwe and Cameroon, that define intellectual disability according to norms of the society they live in. These negative stereotypes in most of the African countries have led to the exclusion of individuals with ID from the mainstream society [21]. This has even led to some families to hide their adolescents allowing them to grow in isolation with no proper transition. It is therefore not surprising that in most of Africa, there is lack of relevant policies for individuals with ID, and this poses many challenges for them and their families. Most of these challenges relate to social, occupational and parental issues.

3.1 Social challenges with transition of adolescents with intellectual disability

Lack of support and labelling of individuals with ID by communities are some of the challenges that affect adolescents with ID. These lead to isolation and loneliness. Other studies [2, 22, 23] also reported that individuals with ID are ridiculed, not supported and unaccepted by the society they live in. Stigma and discrimination, especially in African countries where disability is associated with witchcraft and other supernatural causes, influence the way the individuals with ID are treated. Incidences of individuals with ID being locked in the houses and hidden from the larger society are still rife in some parts of Africa [24].

Adolescents with ID may not even have the opportunity to volunteer for some activities in their communities. Friendships and peer interactions are limited mostly because other peers with no ID may react negatively towards those with ID, and it is because they have differing conceptions of friendships [25].

3.2 Occupational challenges with transition of adolescents with intellectual disabilities

Adolescents with ID face many challenges, especially in developing countries. There are very few schools open to adolescents with ID. The majority of them end at the seventh grade. This is especially true if they come from poor families who may not afford few private schools. In a study by Malapela [26], she found that out of the 25 adolescents admitted in two special schools in South Africa, only one of them was given a vocational job after completion. In other countries, there are social grants with which these individuals and their families depend on, whereas in other countries where there are no disability grants, their livelihood is dependent on their parents and families. Pandey and Agarwal [5] reported that adolescents with ID are most likely not to be employed and less likely to complete secondary education.

3.3 Leisure challenges with transition of adolescents with intellectual disabilities

It is generally believed that leisure promotes emotional and psychological wellbeing for individuals with ID [27]. Leisure activities develop general skills and adaptive behaviours. However, in most countries leisure activities for individuals with ID are limited or non-existent Majoko [28]. Lack of leisure or recreational activities leave the individual with ID to have television as an only option. For some who do not have television, they spend most of the time in the house watching movements of their people depending on the degree of their disability. For some, parents may not allow their adolescents with ID to play with others for fear that they would be hurt, mocked or ridiculed. Jerome, Frantino and Sturmey [29] see this as being overprotective, which does not benefit the individual with ID as taking risks of being hurt is part of growing up. All these are daily challenges faced by these individuals.

3.4 Parental challenges

Literature has reported stress and depression for parents of adolescents with ID. Parents experience caregiver burden because in most cases they are left alone to care for their adolescents with no external assistance. In most instances, the parents are responsible for attending to all the activities of daily living for their adolescents with ID. A study conducted in United Kingdom by Rogers [30] reported that parenting an individual with intellectual disability incapacitates the whole family. It puts more pressure and burden on the family as more attention is needed from parents and mothers of these individuals to assist them to achieve activities of daily living including bathing, feeding, mobility, toilet training, socialising and others. The caregiver burden is aggravated by lack of professional support and unavailability of services. The American Psychological Association (2016) is of the view that where there is support and services the caregiver burden would be lessened. In other countries, where there is absence of such facilities or the lack of knowledge about their existence, then parental stress can be exacerbated [26].

4. Governmental interventions

Transition of adolescents with ID into adulthood has been a concern not just for researchers but for national governments as well. Most governments encourage the principle of inclusion in schools and employment [7]. In some instances, policies have been developed that encourage inclusion and provide more opportunities for adolescents with ID aiming at maximising their interaction with the wider community.

In South Africa, for instance, a number of legislative regulations and policy framework have been developed to protect individuals with intellectual disabilities from exploitation, vulnerability and discrimination. However, numerous concerns and challenges have been reported regarding their care, treatment and rehabilitation that are detrimental to their general wellbeing and their future prospects. According to the policy guidelines on child and adolescent mental health and reconstruction and development programme (RDP), adolescents with ID are still faced by many challenges in their transition to adulthood. It is for this reason that transition possibilities need to be prioritised.

The Mental Health Care Act No.17 of 2002 that directs care, treatment and rehabilitation of adolescents with intellectual disabilities states that individuals with ID have the right to a sheltered employment and fair treatment. However, the demands of this act have not been realised fully, and this impacts negatively on their transition.

Given all the limitations that affect the transition possibilities, proper understanding of transition possibilities in the context of intellectual disabilities needs urgent attention. There must be a change that would have positive impact in the lives of individuals with ID. These changes must take cognisance of their level of mental, physical, social and emotional functioning.

5. Transition possibilities

There are numerous transition possibilities that could be done to assist adolescents with ID. Most of these possibilities centre on what governments and healthcare workers can do to mitigate the many challenges associated with their transitions. The possibilities for governments are on policy development and involvement of other stakeholders. For healthcare workers, the main theme is on educating different players such as parents, families and communities.

6. The role of governments

Poor outcomes for adolescents with ID on employment, education and social activities call for an active path for changing the post high school scenery. Governments can strive to make transition easier by ensuring structures that accommodate adolescents with ID are in place. Firstly, governments should ensure that all the schools from primary to secondary have facilities for special education. Such an arrangement will ensure that adolescents with ID and those without ID are taught in the same schools. Arrangements could be made that in such schools there will exist common courses that are taken together such as physical education. This will have multiple benefits for all. Adolescents with no ID will be able to accept those with ID and can understand their shortcomings and be able to assist them.

Firm friendships can be built at this stage, and this would ensure that adolescents with IDs leisure time are well taken care of [5]. The authors reported that adolescents with ID believe that they are just like others and consider themselves able to interact with peers with no ID. Research by Kurth and Mastergeorge [31] suggest that inclusive education has more enhanced academic results for students with disabilities.

The use of technology in such schools will also improve the academic outcomes for students with ID. Therefore, governments should strive to make all this available for adolescents with ID. Maxey and Beckett [7] posit that special education which is in the same environment with the mainstream education plays a vital role on how adolescents with ID are perceived by both the teachers and their peers. Currently in most countries, especially in developing countries, there are very few special schools, hence governments should be encouraged to build some and make them inclusive.

Governments can also expand employment opportunities for adolescents with ID. These they could do through collaborating with employment agencies. A study done by Plotner and Mashall [32] in the United States found that 28.4% of adults with ID were in formal employment compared to 71% of those adults without ID. However, in developing countries the statistics would even be lower. Adolescents with ID should be taught courses that would link them with particular employment opportunities.

Community centres that are open for adolescents with ID need to be in place. The government can achieve this by forming partnerships with community agencies. The benefit of this would be that it would allow for integration of adolescents with ID into the community. Pallisera et al. [33] argued that transition partnerships and collaboration are key factors in the facilitation and fostering of the transition process. This means an inclusion of a wide range of professionals, agencies, centres or services throughout the transition process.

Healthcare services are fragmented in most countries. For adolescents with ID, this would compound the problem of caregivers; hence, the governments need to bring them together. In most countries there are no services tailored for adolescents. There are health services for children and for adults, and there are very few for adolescents such as youth centres. This gap in service provision should be attended to, and youth-friendly services and skill centres should be made available even for adolescents with ID.

7. The role of healthcare workers

In order to ensure successful healthy transitions in healthcare, partnership work with families, communities, societies, education and other relevant stakeholders is needed. Ramalhal et al. [34] assert that nurses have the responsibility to assist individuals and their families to deal with the transition process. On the contrary, Shaw and DeLaet [12] argue that the physicians should take the first critical step to improve the transition process to adult-oriented healthcare. According to Meleis' Transition Theory, nurses are the partners of individuals and their families as they will be able to follow changes and outcomes regarding the transition process.

Healthcare workers are also responsible for educating parents on the adolescent's condition and what parents should expect. This would lessen the stress and ensure that parents know what to do with their adolescents. Education should focus on the adolescent behaviour. This would help parents to develop healthy relationships with their adolescent. This education should involve not just primary caregivers but extended family such as siblings, grandparents, aunts and other significant parties.

Healthcare workers are also charged with explaining to families about the level and scope of healthcare services that are available for such individuals. In most cases, families get confused because they are not aware of services that are available to adolescents with ID. Healthcare workers can facilitate their formation so that families can support and encourage each other.

Families should also be educated on the importance of a friendly, safe and stimulating environment to enable adolescents with ID to maximise their potentials and to cushion emotional and behavioural challenges [26]. Internet should be used where possible, and computer skills should be developed. Seal [35] and Seal and Pockney [36] hold a strong view that the use of the Internet allows individuals with ID to express themselves.

Provision of counselling is another viable transition possibility [26]. Individuals with ID should be counselled if they get frustrated in their inability to solve problems and be encouraged if they are able to solve problems on their own. Healthcare in most countries is very fragmented; healthcare workers should support their integration so that counselling is offered with other services. This would ensure that individuals with ID receive total quality care when is needed.

In a study by Malapela [26], it was found that the majority of parents lacked the knowledge and skill to care for their adolescents with ID. The study recommended that educating caregivers on the care of their adolescents and knowledge about their limitations would promote positive transition outcomes.

8. The role of communities

Teaching communities and socialisation of the intellectually disabled children into the community are the key factors that form the basis for assisting adolescents with

IDs transition into adulthood. If communities understand the abilities and limitations of adolescents with ID, they would have a nondiscriminatory attitude that would assist in the transition outcomes for individuals with ID. A non-judgemental and nondiscriminatory attitude is key towards achieving healthy transition experience.

Community partnerships with parents and professionals would relieve parents from being alone in the care of their intellectually disabled. Therefore, working together as a team would ensure a healthy transition of individuals with ID. For transition to bring about change and difference, individuals, their families and health and non-healthcare professionals should make necessary efforts and changes that enable these individuals and their families to adapt to their new roles and expectations. A community approach is necessary to assist these individuals, their families and their caregivers adapt to new changes and routines. Therefore, community education is essential to ensure that transition process promote positive experiences.

More community resources should be available and accessible to support these individuals and their families during the transition experience and process.

9. Conclusion

Positive transition of adolescents with ID would ensure improvement of quality of life for individuals with ID. Governments and other stakeholders need to further develop the policy framework needed to assist individuals with ID and related interventions. Education, employment and leisure are key to a fruitful integration of individuals with ID in the mainstream society. Studies quoted in this chapter support those individuals with ID to have the same opportunities as for all individuals without ID. Prioritisation of provision and development of working skills are the determining factors for facilitating transition of adolescents with IDs into adulthood. The need for further research is necessary to ensure that adolescent with ID can live an independent life.

Author details

Rakgadi Grace Malapela* and Gloria Thupayagale-Tshweneagae*
University of South Africa, Pretoria, South Africa

*Address all correspondence to: gmalapela@gmail.com and tshweg@unisa.ac.za

References

[1] Steinberg L. Age of Opportunity: Lessons from the New Science of Adolescence. Boston, MA: Houghton Mifflin Harcourt; 2014

[2] Mudhovozi P, Maphula A, Mashamba T. Caring for children with mental retardation: The experiences of Vhavenda mothers. *African*. Journal for Physical. Health Education. Recreation and Dance (AJPHERD). 2012;**2**:148-159

[3] Nyangweso M. Disability in Africa: A cultural/religious perspective. East Carolina University. ResearchGate.net; 2018

[4] Meleis AI, Sawyer LM, Im EO, Messias DKH, Schumacher K. Experiencing transitions: An emerging middle range theory. Advances in Nursing Science. 2000;**23**(1):12-28

[5] Pandey S, Agarwal S. Transition to adulthood for youth with disability: Issues for the disabled child and family. JOSR Journal of Humanities and Social Science (IOSR-JHSS). 2013;**17**(3):41-45

[6] Foley KR, Dyke P, Bourke J, Leonard H. Young adults with intellectual disability transitioning from school to post-school: A literature review framed within the ICF. Disability and Rehabilitation. 2012;**34**(20):1747-1764

[7] Maxey M, Beckett TE. Adolescents and disabilities. Adolescent Research Review. 2017;**2**:59-75

[8] Malapela G, Mfidi F, Sibanda S, Thupayagale-Tshweneagae G. Caring for mental health care users with profound intellectual disabilities: Approaches and opportunities. Africa Journal of Nursing and Midwifery. 2017;**19**:1-10

[9] Chick N, Meleis AI. Transitions: A nursing concern. In: P.L. Chinn editor. Nursing Research Methodology. Boulder, CO: Aspen; 1986. pp. 237-257

[10] Ally s, Boyd K, Abells D, Amaria K, Hamdani Y, Lo A, et al. Improving transition to adulthood for adolescents with intellectual and developmental disabilities. Canadian Family Physcian. 2018;**64**(2):S37-S43

[11] Ferraioli S, Harris S. The impact of autism on siblings. Social Work in Mental Health. 2010;**8**:41-53

[12] Shaw TM, DeLaet DE. Transition of adolescents to young adulthood for vulnerable populations. Pediatrics in Review. 2010;**31**(12):1-4

[13] Patterson I, Pegg S. Serious leisure and people with intellectual disabilities: Benefits and opportunities. Leisure Studies. 2009;**28**(4):387-402

[14] Foley KR, Taffe J, Bourke J, Einfeld SL, Tonge JT, Leonard H. Young people with intellectual disability transitioning into adulthood: Do behaviour trajectories differ in those with and without down syndrome. PLoS One. 2016;**11**(7):1-9

[15] Aldersey HM. Family perception of intellectual disability: Understanding and support in Dar es Salaam. African Journal of Disability. 2012;**1**(1):32. DOI: 10.4102/ajod.v1i1.32

[16] Werner S. Individuals with intellectual disabilities: A review of the literature on decision-making since the convention on the rights of people with disabilities (CRPD). Public Health Reviews. 2012;**34**(2):1-27

[17] Lancaster RL, Balling K, Hastings R, Lloyd TJ. Attributions, criticism and warmth in mothers of children with intellectual disability and challenging behaviour: A pilot study. Journal of Intellectual Disability Research. 2014;**58**:1060-1071

[18] Shogren KA, Plotner AJ. Transition planning for students with intellectual disability autism or other disabilities: Data from the National Longitudinal. Intellectual and Developmental Disabilities. 2012;**50**(1):16-30

[19] Mckenzie JA, McConkey R, Adnams C. Intellectual disability in Africa: Implications for research and service development. Disability and Rehabilitation. 2013;**35**(20):1750-1755

[20] Etiyiebo E, Omiegbe O. Religion, culture, and discrimination against persons with disabilities in Nigeria. African Journal of Disability. 2016;**5**(1):1-6. DOI: 1o.4102/ajod.v5i1.192

[21] Koszela K. The Stigmatization of Disabilities in Africa and the Development Effects, Independent Study project Collection 1639. 2013. Available from: http://digitalcollections.sit.edu/ISP-collection/1639

[22] Tugli AK, Zungu LI, Ramakuela NJ, Goon DT, FC A. Perceived challenges of serving students with disabilities in a historically disadvantaged tertiary institution, South Africa. African Journal for Physical Health Education. Recreation and Dance (AJPHERD) (Supplement). 2013;**1**(2):346-355

[23] Vermeer A, Magyarszeky Z. Disability Care in Africa Community Based Rehabilitation in Rural Regions. 1st ed. Netherlands, Amsterdam: VU University Press; 2014

[24] Acker J. Inequality regimes: Gender, class, and race in organisations. Gender and Society. 2006;**20**(4):441-464

[25] Rossetti Z. Descriptors of friendship between secondary students with and without autism or intellectual and developmental disability. Remedial and Special Education. 2015;**36**(3):181-192

[26] Malapela RG. Strategy for transition of adolescents with intellectual disabilities into adulthood (thesis). Pretoria, SA: University of South Africa; 2018

[27] Buttimer J, Tiery E. Patterns of leisure participation among adolescents with mild intellectual disability. Journal of Intellectual Disabilities. 2005;**9**(1):25-42

[28] Majoko T. Inclusion of children with disabilities in physical education in Zimbabwean primary schools. SAGE Open. 2019;**8**:1-16

[29] Jerome J, Frantino EP, Sturmey P. The effects of errorless learning and backward chaining on the acquisition of Internet skills in adult with developmental disabilities. Journal of Applied Behaviour Analysis. 2007;**40**(1):185-189

[30] Rogers C. Mothering and intellectual disability: Partnership rhetoric? British Journal of Sociology of Education. 2011;**32**(4):563-581

[31] Kurth JA, Mastergeorge AM. Individual education plan goals and services for adolescents with autism: Impact of age and educational setting. Journal of Special Education. 2010;**44**:146-160

[32] Plotner AJ, Marshall KJ. Supporting post-secondary education programs for individuals with an intellectual disability: Role of the vocational rehabilitation counselor. Institute on Disabilities Hammill. 2016;**59**(4):195-202

[33] Pallisera M, Vila M, Fullana J. Transition to adulthood for young people with intellectual disability: Exploring transition partnerships from the point of view of professionals in school and post school services. Journal of Intellectual and Developmental Disability. 2014;**3**(4):333-341

[34] Ramalhal T, Lagarto A, Matos A, Cruz H, Ribeiro H. Transition to parenthood: Nursing intervention to promote paternal competences. NERP. 2013;**5**:164-169

[35] Seale JK. The same but different: The use of the personal home page by adults with down syndrome as a tool for self-presentation. British Journal of Educational Technology. 2001;**32**: 343-352. DOI: 10.1111/1467-8535.00203

[36] Seale JK, Pockney R. The use of the personal home page by adults with down syndrome as a tool for managing identity and friendship. British Journal of Learning Disabilities. 2002;**30**:142-148. DOI: 10.1046/j.1468-3156.2002.00195.x

Chapter 13

Speech Therapy Work with Children Having Specific Language Impairment: Algorithms and Personalization

Tatiana Volodarovna Tumanova
and Tatiana Borisovna Filicheva

Abstract

The concept of "personalization" is rather strengthened in pedagogy. At the same time, in Russia in the field of special pedagogy and, in particular, in speech therapy, there is an urgent need for personalized influence with specific language impairments. A review of Russian classical and modern data on the comorbidity of speech, language, motor skills, and other processes in children with specific language disorders is presented. The rationale for personifying speech therapy work in children with specific language impairments was justified. The scientific positions of the authors with respect to personalization in the field of differential evaluation, developmental effects, and prevention of systemic consequences of specific language impairments in children are indicated. The groups of personalized means and aids of influence of a speech therapist for specific language impairments in children are indicated. The directions of further development of the indicated problem of personalization of speech therapy work are determined.

Keywords: personalization, children of preschool age, personalized means and aids of speech therapy work, specific language impairment in children, personalized diagnostic profile, comorbidity of speech, language and motor disorders

1. Introduction

In world science, and in Russian speech therapy, in particular, the issues of differential evaluation and in-depth study of specific language disorders in children are dynamically developing [1–3]. The manifestations and symptoms revealed by the authors determine the understanding of the underlying mechanisms of such a state as "specific language impairment." This allows to study in detail the structure of impaired development, to determine strategies and directions of developmental effects of speech therapy. Therefore, in Russian science, the search for further ways of a transdisciplinary study of the problem of helping children with SLI remains very relevant in special pedagogy in general, and speech therapy, in particular. It can be stated that in modern speech therapy, as a science, it is defined as a number of contradictions. On the one hand, there is a need to find new and improving existing approaches to the speech therapy work with children with SLI. On the other hand methodological, substantive, organizational, and other aspects of new and modernized approaches to solving the designated problem are insufficiently developed. The resolution of the existing contradictions, of course, occurs, and will continue to take place in scientific research of several generations. However, today, we can say that a personalized approach in speech therapy work with SLI children meets the abovementioned social challenges and contributes to effectively overcoming pressing contradictions in general, inclusive, and special education.

In Russian pedagogy, interest in the development of a personalized approach can be traced in the writings of scientists starting last century [1]. There are different interpretations of personalization in education, which allows interpreting this phenomenon in different ways. Personalization can be explained as the process of gaining by a subject universal human, socially significant, individually unique properties and qualities that allow him to fulfill a certain social role in an original way, creatively build communication with other people, and actively influence their perception and assessment of their own personality and activities [2]. At the same time, the term "personalization in education" is often used in Russian scientific research, interpreted extremely variably as: a special form of organization of the educational process, taking into account the peculiarities of personal differences of students [3]; one of the directions of modernization of the system of continuous education; a process aimed at the development of students' abilities and interests [4]; a factor of development of cognitive activity of trainees; and a means of building a personal educational route [5]. The personalization of education is also considered as a didactic principle, according to which the content and all other elements of the educational process should be determined and built on the basis of the interests, needs, and aspirations of persons involved in educational activities [6].

The variability of interpretations, however, reflects the general focus of educational processes in Russia on the dynamic development of such pedagogical paradigms that put the student's personality and his multidirectional interests and needs at the center of pedagogical processes.

Moreover, the relevance of a personalized approach in the field of evaluation and development work of a speech therapist with SLI children seems logical.

2. Speech therapy impact at SLI in Russia: algorithms or personalization?

For many decades, Russia has developed stable algorithms for speech therapists: how to work with children with specific language impairments. Those algorithms are based on the classic Russian level approach to assessing the linguistic and speech status of such children [7]. For many decades (since the 60s of the last century), Russian speech therapy has developed an understanding of the essence of SLI as a developmental speech\language disorder that has signs of systemic underdevelopment of all language components and embraces all speech processes [8]. In this regard, in Russia, national models for evaluation of children with SLI have been identified and are successfully operating to date. These models bring together an interdisciplinary team of specialists, which conducts a comprehensive examination of children, evaluates the state of various functions, and formulates a conclusion and recommendations for working with a particular child (psychologist, pediatrician, neurologist, speech therapist, teacher-representative of the school, and if necessary, other specialists). The speech therapist as part of this team conducts his assessment. It can be variable in technology and didactic materials, but always includes: collecting data on the development of language and speech of the child and the speech environment in his family, understanding of speech and language structures, the state of vocabulary, grammar, phonetics, dialogical and monologue utterances (in relation to the age indicators of normative development). The diagnostic program also includes examination of the state of operations of language analysis and synthesis (starting from 3 to 4 years of age), the state of the basics of literacy (from 6 years old), and later (from 7 to 8 years) an examination is added to the above writing, reading, counting operations, and other educational skills. For many decades, scientific research data, covering various regions of Russia, confirmed the idea of professor R.E. Levina, and, later, professor T.B. Filicheva that the speech-language status of children with SLI can be understood as very different, varying within different levels: from the first level (lowest) to the fourth level (somewhat close to the lower limits of the age norm) [7–9]. The national practice of speech therapy allows detecting a delay in the development of speech/language in children from 2 to 3 years of age with a normative state of intelligence and hearing, in order to subsequently consider these children as a risk group for detecting SLI in them, starting from 3 years. Accordingly, it is from this age in Russia that it is customary to designate a condition revealed in a child not as delayed, but as a disordered development of language and speech. The context of this approach is reflected in the national psycho-pedagogical classification of speech\ language disorders [9]. In Russian speech therapy, a hierarchy of short level characteristics has been established that testifies to the underdevelopment of the processes of language and speech in children with SLI, starting from the age of three:

- *The first level* characterizes practically nonspeaking children who understand the extremely limited volume of words. They use single simple words, amorphous root words, sound complexes, and parts of words, sounds associated with what is named, not combining them into a phrase. There are no word endings, understanding and use of prepositions is not observed. Word formation is not available. A child cannot compose a story on his own. Monological speech is practically absent. A dialogue with such a child shows his active use of nonverbal means of communication. The phonetic side of speech is significantly disturbed; sounds from different phonetic groups are not formed. Children do not understand the tasks aimed at distinguishing the verbal sounds.

- *The second level*—the beginning of the sentence development: children begin to combine two or three words into a simple sentence. However, these sentences are characterized by violations of structure and content. Understanding of speech lags significantly behind these normotypic children. Children skip or distort prepositions, as well as morphemic parts of words, which allow differentially denoting the number, size, gender of objects, objects actions and signs, and other categorical qualities. The initial attempts to form words with significant structural and substantive errors may manifest. Children enter into a dialogue, but do not initiate it, rather respond in one or two words. There is still a tendency to use nonverbal means of communication. Children cannot talk about events, retell the text, etc. Tasks related to distinguishing the verbal sounds are not feasible. The pronunciation of different groups of sounds is characterized by multiple violations.

- *The third level* characterizes using a simple sentence with multiple lexical and grammatical errors. For children at the third level, it becomes possible to draw up simple and even some types of complicated sentences. Nevertheless, in these sentences, there are obvious errors: omissions and rearrangement of the order of the sentence parts, replacement of the end of words, replacement of prepositions, multiple lexical changes and errors (e.g., according to the genus-specific characteristics of words). Children can actively engage in dialogue, but there is a steady tendency toward a passive role. Self-compilation of the story, retelling of the text, becomes possible. At the same time, expressed errors are allowed in the transmission of the text, its composition, cause and effect, logical and temporal relationships. Word formation and change of words by grammatical categories is characterized by persistent, constant errors (choice of morpheme, choice of grammatical model, word design, etc.). The ability to distinguish some sounds of the native language appears. However, sounding phonemes do not differentiate as should be in accordance with the age of children. They found disturbed pronunciation of sounds from different phonetic groups.

- *The fourth level* characterizes residual manifestations of mildly expressed underdevelopment of vocabulary, grammar, phonetics, and storytelling. Single, but persistent manifestations of impaired development of language and speech are noted in almost all areas, but as minimal manifestations. Such micro-manifestations in the underdevelopment of speech and language, however, are systemic. They show the need for further continuation of the work of the speech therapist [8, 10].

These characteristics of the level assessment of the state of speech and language in children, on the one hand, represent an algorithmized understanding of the fact that underdevelopment of the studied processes of varying severity can be observed in SLI. However, on the other hand, this approach already determines personalization in assessing the language and speech of a child with SLI (if there are common characteristics of underdevelopment inherent in one or another level). The speech-language data of each child are compared with indicators of the age norm. At the same time, indicators of insufficient development of language and speech inherent in each specific child are revealed. In accordance with such a layered approach, confirmed by hundreds of scientific studies and many decades of scientific and practical work, speech therapists in Russia successfully perfect effective algorithms for optimal care for children with SLI. These algorithms are based on determining the level of development of language and speech capabilities that correspond to the current state of the child, and the level that is promising and achievable for him in the course of development work, taking into account the social needs of the child [8, 10, 11].

Currently, these speech therapist work algorithms are reflected in training programs for children with SLI (e.g., programs for overcoming SLI in preschool children) [12].

Such training programs for children offer speech therapists a simple and transparent algorithm of work. It includes a plan for working with a child (with first, second, third, or fourth level of underdevelopment of speech-language processes), the content of the work, the main guidelines for the formation of the lexical, grammatical, phonetic, and syntactic possibilities of children, as well as the potential results that the speech therapist seeks in his work.

So, in working with children whose level of speech and language capabilities is assessed as the minimum (*first level*), the speech therapy is aimed at:

- development of understanding of speech: to teach according to the instructions of a speech therapist to recognize and show objects, actions, signs, understand the generalizing meaning of a word, differentially perceive who and where, and understand appeal to one or more persons, grammatical categories of the number of nouns, verbs, guess objects according to their description, determine elementary cause-effect relationships;

- the development of active speech activity: in any phonetic design, to name parents, close relatives, imitate the cries of animals and birds, sounds of the world, musical instruments; give orders—go, sit, give; make up the first sentences from amorphous root words (*mama pi*—mama, go to sleep), convert imperative verbs into singular verbs of the present tense, make sentences according to the model: (a) Who? what does? (b) Who? what does? what? (e.g., Katia (mom, dad) is sleeping; Anna drinks milk). Simultaneously, exercises are conducted to develop memory, attention, logical thinking (remembering 2–4 objects, guessing the removed or added object, remembering and selecting pictures of 2–4 parts).

As a result of speech therapy work at this stage of the formation of speech\language development, children learn to correlate objects and actions with their verbal designation, to understand the general meaning of words. An active and passive dictionary should consist of the names of objects that the child often sees; actions performed by himself or others, of some of his states (cold, warm). Children need to communicate with the help of elementary two-three-word sentences. Verbal activity can be manifested in any phrases without correction of their phonetic design.

Teaching children with a *second level* of speech/language development involves several areas:

- development of understanding of speech: includes the formation of the ability to listen to the converted speech, to highlight the names of objects, actions, and some signs; the formation of understanding the generalized meaning of words; and preparation for the perception of dialogical and monological speech.

- activation of speech activity and the development of lexical and grammatical means of the language: learn to name words made up of one to three syllables (cat, bed, coat, puppy), teach initial inflection skills, then derivation (number of nouns, mood and number of verbs, possessive pronouns "my—mine," nouns with diminutive suffixes, categories of case of nouns).

- development of active phrase: construction and use models of simple sentences—noun plus a coordinated verb in the indicative mood of the singular present tense, noun plus a coordinated verb in the indicative mood of the singular present tense plus a noun in the indirect case (of type "Misha, sleep," "Misha is sleeping," "Lilia drinks milk"); assimilation of simple prepositions—on, at, in; combining simple sentences into short stories; strengthen the skills of drawing up proposals for demonstrating actions based on questions; memorization of short couplets and nursery rhymes. Moreover, any phonetic design of independent expressions available to the child is allowed, while attention is paid to the correct grammatically significant elements (endings, suffixes, etc.).

- development of the pronunciation: to learn to distinguish between speech and nonspeech sounds to determine the source, strength, and direction of sound; to clarify the correct pronunciation of the sounds available to the child; develop the sounds at the level of the syllables, of the sentence, words, form the correct sound-syllabic structure of the word; to learn to distinguish and reproduce clearly syllabic combinations of sounds with different stresses, voice strength, and intonation; and play the syllables with a concourse of consonants.

As a result of speech therapy work by the end of this stage of education, children should have a simple phrase, learn to coordinate the main parts of a sentence, understand and use simple prepositions, categories of case, number, time, and gender. The ability to answer questions with a short sentence, to maintain dialogue, is supposed. The understanding of some grammatical forms of words, simple stories, short tales is expanded. Work on the syllabic structure of words ends with the assimilation of the rhythmic-syllable pattern of two-syllable and three-syllable words. Sound disturbances are permissible.

Education for children with a *third level* of speech/language development includes:

- the development of speech understanding, the ability to listen to the speech addressed to person, to differentially perceive the names of objects, the actions of signs; to develop an understanding of more subtle meanings of generalizing words, to prepare for mastering monologic and dialogical speech.

- the formation of the phonetic system of the language:

(a) the development of the ability to differentiate listening oppositional speech sounds: whistling-hissing, voiced-deaf, hard-soft, etc., then, working out these differentiations in pronunciation; (b) consolidation of the pronunciation of polysyllabic words with various variants of the concordance of consonants, the use of these words in speech; (c) strengthening the skills of sound analysis and synthesis (analysis and synthesis of a simple syllable without consonants, emphasis on the initial vowel/consonant in a word, analysis and synthesis of syllables with confluence of consonants, emphasis on the final consonant/vowel in a word, division of a word into syllables, analysis and synthesis of 2-compound words, etc.).

- literacy training: acquaintance with letters corresponding to correctly pronounced sounds; learning the elements of sound-alphanumeric analysis and synthesis when working with syllable and word schemes; read and write single syllables, words, and short sentences. Preparation for mastering elementary writing and reading skills includes consolidating the concepts of "sound," "syllable," "word," "sentence," "story," analysis and synthesis of sound-syllabic and sound-alphabetic structures.

- the development of lexical and grammatical means of language. This section includes not only an increase in quantitative, but primarily qualitative indicators: the expansion of the meanings of words; the formation of the semantic structure of the word; the introduction of new words and phrases into speech of nouns with a diminutive and magnifying meaning, with the opposite meaning. The ability to explain the figurative meaning of words (golden hands, sharp tongue etc.). Select unambiguous nouns for adjectives (sharp—knife, sauce, razor, seasoning; dark—shawl, night, coat); form names of objects from the action names; explain logical connections (Nata escorted Sofia—who came?), to pick up synonyms (bold—brave).

- the development of detailed phrasal speech phonetically correctly formed; formation of dialogue skills; expanding the skills of composing a narrative story based on the events of a given sequence, drawing up sentences with different types of subordinate clauses, strengthening the ability to compose stories from a picture, a series of paintings, by presentation, by demonstrating actions, transforming a deformed text; and the inclusion in the stories of the beginning and end of the plot, elements of fantasy.

As a result of speech therapy work children should master the skills of using simple and complex sentences, be able to take part in dialogue; be able to compose a story from a picture and a series of pictures, retell the text, have a grammatically correct spoken language in accordance with the basic norms of the language; it is phonetically correct to make statements, conveying the syllabic structure of words, to master some elements of literacy (reading and typing letters, syllables, and short words). However, they may have some lexical, grammatical, and phonetic inaccuracies, the elimination of which should be combined with teaching children complex forms of speech, which is proposed to be done at the next stage of training.

Teaching children with the *fourth level* of speech\language development provides areas of work related to their comprehensive preparation for school:

- Improvement of the lexical and grammatical means of the language: expansion of the lexical stock in the process of learning new words and lexical groups (shell, tusks, museum, theater, exhibition etc.), activation of word-formation processes (complex words, adjectives with different correlation values, prefixes with tinted values), exercise in the selection of synonyms, and antonyms, giving them explanations (mean—greedy, kind—merciful, funny—sad, etc.), explain the figurative expression of words and whole expressions (burn with shame, wide soul), transform the names of male professions' gender into feminine names (typical for Russian), and convert one grammatical category into another (read—reader).

- Development of phrasal speech: to consolidate the skill of using sentences in reference words, to expand the volume of sentences by introducing homogeneous members of sentences.

- Improve coherent statements, ability to build dialogue and monologue, reinforce storytelling skills, retelling with elements of fantasy and creative stories.

- Improvement of the pronunciation in speech: to consolidate the skills of clear pronunciation and distinguishing of delivered sounds, automate their correct pronunciation in polysyllabic words and statements, to bring up the rhythmic and melodic coloring of speech.

- Preparation for mastering elementary writing and reading skills: reinforce the concepts of "sound," "syllable," "word," "sentence," learn to analyze and synthesize reverse and direct syllables and monosyllables—two, three complex words, learn to make letters, split alphabet, syllables, words and read them, develop optical-spatial and motor-graphic skills, and prepare for a fluent sequential reading with awareness of the meaning of what was read.

As a result of speech therapy, preschool children should be as close as possible to age norms. This is manifested in the spontaneous, faultless possession of dialogical and monologue speech, namely: the ability to adequately formulate questions and answer the questions of others, to tell in detail and logically about the events of the real world, to retell literary texts close to the original, carry out creative storytelling, etc. Accordingly, the lexical and grammatical structure of the language is formed in children. So, children adequately understand and use the various parts of speech, simple and complex prepositions, possess the full knowledge of word formation and inflection for the full extent specified for the specified age. The phonetic design of children's speech should fully comply with the norms of their native language. In addition, children have sufficiently formed operations of sound-syllabic analysis and synthesis and elementary literacy skills (reading and typing some letters, syllables, short words) [7].

3. Methodology

The material below is aimed at achieving the goal: to identify personalization opportunities in working with children with SLI. It is traditionally considered that algorithms of speech therapy with SLI take into account an individual approach to working with children. The individual approach is an important psychological and pedagogical principle, according to which the educational characteristics of children take into account the individual characteristics of the development of each child (psychological features, abilities, psychological characteristics, the child's perception of the impact on him, etc.) [13]. In the context of speech therapy work with SLI children, a personalized approach is an equally important principle according to which medical, psychological, pedagogical, and social markers and criteria for their impaired development are taken into account in working with each child from the standpoint of further prediction and implementation of optimally effective speech therapy. With this understanding of the problem, there is no equal sign between the individual and personalized approaches in speech therapy work with SLI children. The need for a holistic algorithm-based work with these children is determined to reasonably take into account the combination of individual and personalized approaches [10, 11, 14].

Russian studies in this area show the variable correlation of the speech-language capabilities of SLI children with emotional-volitional, communicative, motor, spatial-orienting, visual (as later acquired) disorders [10, 11, 14, 15]. For example, the data of recent years allow to speak about the multi-level comorbidity of symptoms and components (in the context of the codependence of impaired speech, language, motor, and other processes) in children with language disorders [16–18]. The levels of comorbidity states identified in preschool children with SLI were determined (based on the results of the analysis of data from a survey of language, speech, motor, optical-spatial, graphic processes). The level of micro-comorbidity is characterized by a slightly pronounced correlation of motor and speech\language disorders with the relative safety of spatial possibilities. The level of meso-comorbidity indicates a persistent, pronounced correlation of violations of speech-language processes (intonation, prosodic, pronunciation, phonological, lexical-grammatical) and motor sphere (myofunctional and motility of the fingers) along with partial violation of spatial possibilities. The level of macro-comorbidity characterizes stable, systemic combination and pronounced correlation of manifestations of speech\language disorders covering all speech processes and language components, and motor disorders covering differentiated myofunctional abilities and movements in the shoulder girdle, hands, and fingers with the accompanying pronounced impairment of spatial capabilities [16, 17]. Below is a summary data illustrating the phenomena of comorbidity in children with SLI (**Table 1**).

All of the above allow us to draw a number of conclusions that are fundamentally important for the personalization of speech therapist work with SLI children as part of an interdisciplinary team of specialists:

- in children with SLI, violations of the development of not only speech and language, but also other processes (motor, spatial and other) are detected;
- manifestations of the severity of these disturbed processes and their compatibility can be variable for each child;

Levels of comorbidity states	Presence of conjugate/codependent violations
Level of micro-comorbidity	Insignificant degree of correlation of violations of pronunciation and distinction of sounds, weak correlation of indicators of reduced understanding of the lexical and grammatical meanings of words and their use in self-expression mainly with indicators of violations of articulation, weak correlation between indicators of impaired speech, language processes and movements of fingers, wrists, shoulder girdle; spatial gnosis and praxis relatively preserved.
Level of meso-comorbidity	Pronounced correlation of speech language processes (intonation, prosodic, pronunciation, phonological, lexical and grammatical) correlating with the indices of motor sphere insufficiency (myofunctional and motility of fingers, wrists etc.) along with partial violation of spatial gnosis and praxis.
Level of macro-comorbidity	Systemic combination and confidently pronounced persistent correlation of manifestations of speech-language impairments, covering all speech processes and components of the language, and motor impairments, covering differentiated myofunctional abilities and movements in the shoulder girdle, hands, and fingers with associated pronounced disorders of spatial gnosis and praxis.

Table 1.
Characteristics of comorbidity levels of speech-language and motor-spatial capabilities of preschool children (5–6 years).

- in this regard, the identification of personal indicators and characteristics of processes disturbed in a child (linguistic, speech, motor, spatial and others) will determine the need for personalization in working with each SLI child, including not only a speech therapist, school teacher, psychologist in the multidisciplinary team, but also other potentially necessary specialists.

All of the above allows to determine the subject of study: the search for reasonable personalized directions, content, means, aids, technologies for working with SLI children.

Between 2010 and 2018 at Moscow State Pedagogical University (Russia, Moscow), the authors conducted a study that covered 460 children with SLI 5–6 years of age, attending educational institutions and receiving the help of a speech therapist using algorithmic educational programs adopted in Russia. These were children whose state of language and speech was assigned to the third level out of four possible levels (according to the national assessment model). At the same time, among the population of children selected for the experiment, half had visual impairment (myopia or strabismus). This led to the formation of two experimental groups—group 1 (230 children with SLI and with good vision) and group 2 (230 children with SLI and impaired vision). For both experimental groups, an examination that combined the following methods was applied:

- standardized examination of language and speech used by speech therapists in Russia (the scheme of this examination was indicated above, the results were recorded in individual protocols for each child);

- diagnosis of the state of movements of the shoulder girdle and fingers according to indicators of completeness, strength, coordination, etc. using Pablo System technology (the results were recorded in individual electronic protocols provided by the software);

- diagnostics of the state of mobility, balance, and coordination using Habilect technology according to the criteria of maintaining equilibrium, coordination of movements of the upper and lower extremities, occupancy, stability of movement, etc. (the results were recorded in individual electronic protocols provided by the software).

For children of the second group (SLI and visual impairment), ophthalmologists were additionally involved in the examination, who for each child gave a professional opinion (on the presence of myopia or strabismus) and formulated recommendations for the teachers' work: what conditions, exercises, and aids are needed for each child, depending on state of his vision.

4. Results

A comparative analysis of the protocols for examining children in the areas outlined above made it possible to personally assess for each child with SLI the starting state of language, speech, motor, and spatial processes. For the second group (children with SLI and visual impairment), ophthalmologists added personal data on the state of visual functions. Thus, as a result, for each child with SLI, a database of linguistic, speech, motor, and visual (for the second group) processes was collected and analyzed. This information is reflected in personal diagnostic profiles, examples of which are given below (**Figures 1–3**).

Figure 1 illustrates a piece of data reflecting part of the overall assessment procedure: the assessment of the quality of statements and stories of a child with SLI and myopia (with\without using of personalized supports) in tasks: No. 1—making a simple sentence based on 1 picture, No. 2—making a simple sentence based on 2 pictures, No. 3—making a simple sentence based on verbal help, No. 4—compiling a story based on a picture, No. 5—composing a story based on a series of paintings, No. 6—composing a story based on verbal help, No. 7—composing a creative story based on a picture. Studies have confirmed that the use of personalized supports when working with a speech therapist with such children gives a pronounced positive effect already at the initial stages of training. The work of a speech therapist for a long time with a child with SLI is all the more effective, provided that in the general algorithm of work those personalized aids and technologies are used

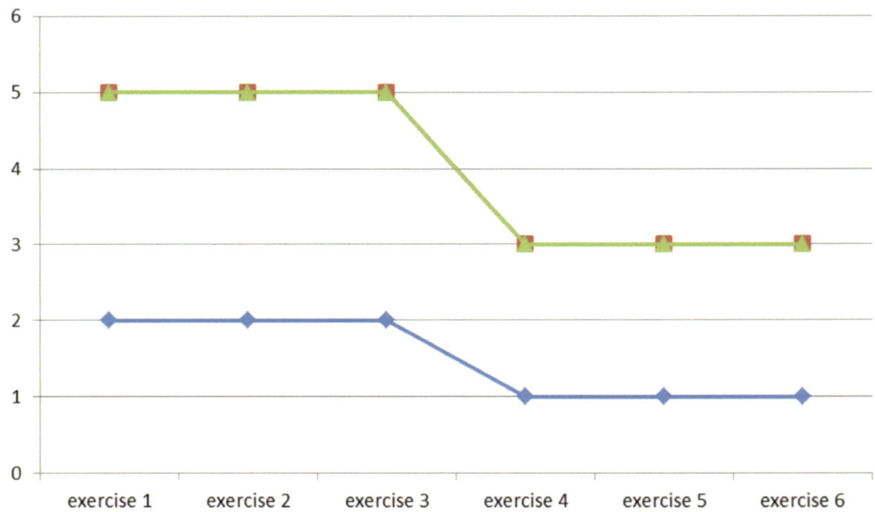

Figure 1.
The profile of the state of connected statements of a child 1 (SLI and myopia) with\without the use of personalized support at the stage of primary linguistic diagnostic procedures.

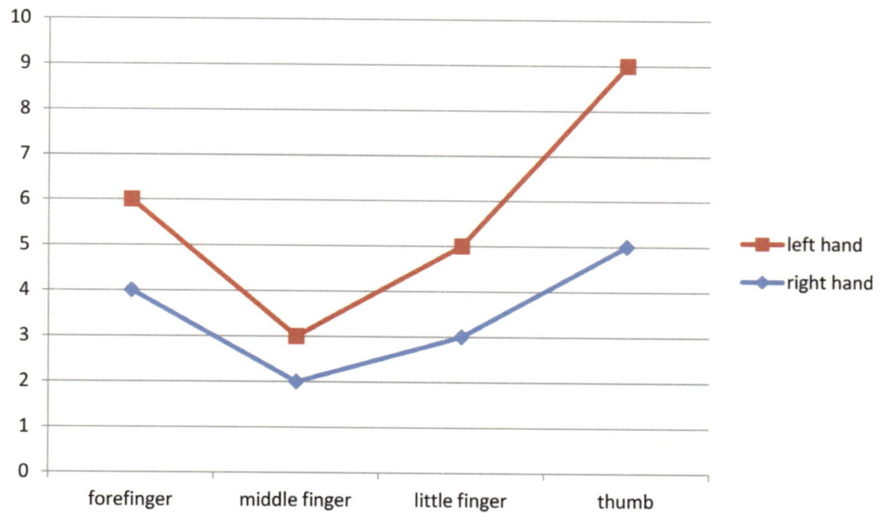

Figure 2.
Two-finger grip state indicators (right and left hand) of a child 1 (SLI and myopia).

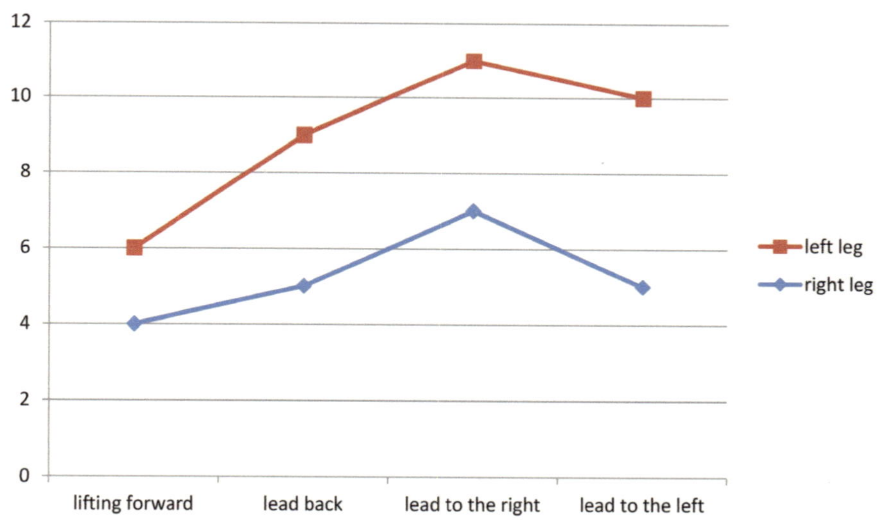

Figure 3.
Indicators of movements of the right/left leg of a child 1 (SLI and myopia).

that help the child with a particular comorbid state of impaired linguistic, motor, spatial, and other processes.

Figure 2 shows a piece of the personal data of child 1 according to the indicators of two-finger pinch capture (right and left hands), demonstrating how accurately and strongly the sensor is captured by different fingers.

Figure 3 shows a piece of the personal data of child 1 on the indicators of leg movements forward, backward, right, and left (right and left legs), showing how accurately and fully the movements are made.

A generalized analysis of the data for each child with SLI has become the basis for planning and implementing personalized exposure programs, designed for 1 year (divided by month and week), for a speech therapist as a member of an interdisciplinary team of specialists. The speech therapist compiled a work plan, based primarily on what starting indicators are recorded in the child in

No	Theme of the lesson	The purpose of the lesson
Week 1		
1	Singular and plural nouns	Learn to use singular and plural nouns
2	Singular and plural nouns	Continue to learn to use singular and plural nouns
3	Word and sentence	To teach to understand and use the concepts of "word," "sentence"
4	Sounds of speech	To teach to understand and use the concept of "Speech Sounds," to distinguish speech sounds from nonspeech
5	Simple sentences	To strengthen the skills of compiling and understanding simple common sentences
Week 2		
1	Verbs singular and plural	Learn to change verbs in the singular and plural categories
2	Verbs singular and plural	Continue learning to change verbs in the singular and plural categories
3	Simple sentences	To strengthen the skills of compiling and understanding simple common sentences
4	Vowels (A, U)	To strengthen the skills of distinguishing and pronunciation of sounds "A-U"
5	Vowels (O)	To strengthen the skills of distinguishing and pronunciation of sound "O"
Week 3		
1	Nouns with a diminutive meaning	To learn to form and use nouns with a diminutive meaning
2	The phrase "quality adjective + noun"	To learn to select and coordinate quality adjectives with nouns
3	Model sentence: Who? What doing?	To strengthen the skills of making sentences on the model of "Who? What doing?"
4	Preposition "on"	To strengthen the skills of distinguishing and pronunciation of preposition "on"
5	Consonant sounds	To strengthen the skills of distinguishing and consonant sounds (1-2 consonants, the most accessible for the child)
Week 4		
1	Nouns with a diminutive meaning	To learn to form and use nouns with a diminutive meaning
2	Model sentence: Who? What doing?	To strengthen the skills of making sentences on the model of: "Who? What doing?"
3	Model sentence: Who? What doing? Where?	To strengthen the skills of making sentences on the model of: "Who? What doing? Where?"
4	Preposition "in"	To strengthen the skills of distinguishing and pronunciation of preposition "in"
5	Consonant sounds (P-B)	Clarify the pronunciation and distinction of sounds "P-B"

Table 2.
A fragment of the sample work plan of a speech therapist with a child 1.

language, speech processes. An exemplary fragment of such planning is shown below (**Table 2**).

However, this plan included areas of work for the development shoulder girdle, finger movements, body movements, leg mobility, as well as those exercises that the ophthalmologist recommended for training the visual muscles. Accordingly, all these exercises were performed by the child either in the process of linguistic tasks, or as independent trainings as a dynamic lesson fragment (using the technologies of Pablo System and Habilect, according to the plan designed by the program of these hardware-computer technologies). "Gymnastics for the eyes" took 2–3 minutes during each lesson and, according to the recommendations of the ophthalmologist, was an obligatory part of the lesson for those children who had visual impairments. Other teachers of the school (physical education teacher, music teacher, and drawing teacher) in their plan of work with each child made personal, substantive, and technological changes based on what were the personal capabilities and needs of each child. The clearly planned work allowed each specialist to carry out his functions, but this was done in mandatory coordination between all team members. In addition to personalizing the content and areas of work, personalized tools and technologies were identified that increase the effectiveness of the speech therapist working with SLI child.

Figure 4 shows the personal data of child 1 obtained when assessing linguistic, speech, motor, and spatial processes primarily (relative to age norm data), and reflects the constancy and stability of the mistakes made when performing language, speech, and motor-spatial tests. **Figure 4** demonstrates the improvement in the child's performance under the condition of a single administration of personalized aids. After provided prolonged (14 weeks) personalized assistance from an interdisciplinary team of specialists, the improvement in the results of child 1 was clearly shown. After each prolonged period of personalized training, a team of specialists discussed the results, drafted amendments and changes to the content, technologies and auxiliary means of working with SLI child. Typically, in speech therapy for SLI, algorithmic exposure programs involve 2 years of training for children with a third level of speech and language development before they reach the next, fourth, level of language development.

At the end of the school year, the results of personalized work with children involved in experimental groups (E group 1—SLI, E group 2—SLI and visual impairment) were analyzed. Each child passed the final assessment according to the same parameters and criteria as before personalized learning. The linguistic and speech processes of all children in the experimental groups turned out to be much higher than at the beginning of the year in all assessment parameters. According to the national model for assessing language and speech status, almost

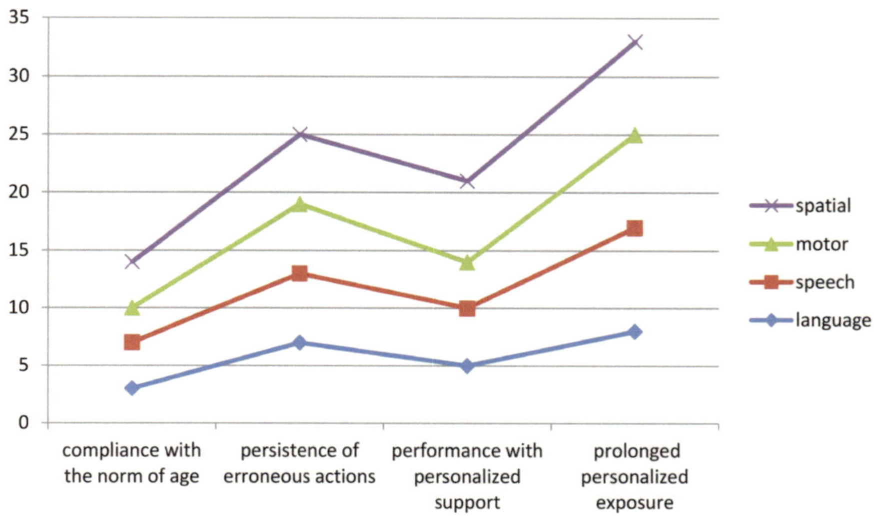

Figure 4.
Generalized indicators of process evaluation of a child 1 (SLI and myopia).

Language development level (according to the national model)	E group 1		E group 2		CA group 1		CA group 2	
	pre	post	pre	post	pre	post	pre	post
Level III	100	20	100	22	100	72	100	82
Level IV	0	80	0	87	0	28	0	18

Table 3.
Analysis of language development data for children with SLI involved in experimental and comparative groups (pre- and post-training) (%).

all children have been changed status from third to fourth level. At the same time, the comparative analysis groups (CA groups), which included children of a similar age who received the work of a speech therapist according to standard exposure algorithms (CA group 1—SLI, CA group 2—SLI and visual impairment) in most cases remained at the third level of speech\language development (**Table 3**).

Table 3 shows data that convincingly show that in the vast majority of cases, the dynamics of language development are higher in those children with ALS who were trained according to personalized programs.

Motor and spatial assessment data using Pablo System and Habilect technologies recorded a personal dynamics for each child, reflecting an improvement in the state of mobility, coordination, strength, motor control in the fingers, wrists, elbow, shoulder, as well as in the movements and coordination of the trunk and legs. The ophthalmologist's data for children with SLI and visual impairments showed varied dynamics (mainly from stabilization of indicators to their slight improvement—81%). The remaining 19% of cases were characterized by an ophthalmologist as a "progressive" course of visual impairment.

5. Discussion

Such data on the impact of personalized teaching aids, which have multiple reproducibility in the study of children with SLI in Russia, subsequently provide weighty reasons for substantial optimization of general, particular, and specific algorithms of speech therapy and developmental influence. At the same time, a personalized approach to it should be understood as a harmonious component of the general scientific and methodological support of the holistic process of psychological and pedagogical assistance for specific language impairment. The effectiveness of this approach seems to be optimal when the following conditions are met: reasonable integration with other approaches strengthened in science and practice, competent use of classical and modern scientific data from the field of speech therapy and related sciences, taking into account variable and combinatorial components in the structure of SLI, based on understanding personalized needs and capabilities of children, the relationship in the interdisciplinary team. The personalization of speech therapy is advisable on the planning and implementation of the content and directions of work, the choice of aids and technologies of influence, logical interaction with other members of the interdisciplinary team.

It is possible to clarify the interpretation of the concept of "personalized aids that ensure the effectiveness of speech therapy work in children with SLI" as a system of various ideal and material objects, including artificially created ones, in order to optimally form language and speech processes in children, as carriers of the necessary information and as instrument. They are integrated at the linguodidactic, logical-semantic, optico-ophthalmological (as prescribed by the ophthalmologist), motor-spatial, and information-technological levels of the problem under study. It is logical to believe that personalization will be in demand in the work of a speech therapist as part of an interdisciplinary team.

Let us consider, for example, the personalization of the content and means of speech therapy work with schoolchildren with SLI and visual impairment (squint and myopia) in the direction associated with the improvement of their coherent expressions. The content of this speech therapy area is traditionally algorithm-driven, based on the appropriate techniques adopted in speech therapy. In parallel, in the context of the joint work of a speech therapist, parents, teachers of physical culture, music, drawing, an ophthalmologist, personalized exercise programs were developed and implemented for such children (depending on the states of comorbidity of speech-language, spatial, optical and motor processes identified for each child) as well as personal plans to perform special visual exercises and workouts. These directions of speech therapy may be changed in content due to child visual impairment. So, in Russian speech therapy, usually a story-description of an object is one of the first forms of work in teaching SLI child storytelling. However, for a child with SLI and visual impairment, we can built a different algorithm that combines analysis and construction: a simple sentence—a fragmentary/holistic dialogue—a narrative story—a descriptive story—a creative story (all types of work are based on a special interactive touch panel with elements of feedback

Groups of personalized aids	Characteristics of aids
Lingvodidactic	Aids that are designed to teach children who have SLI (means to ensure optimal motivation to express, generate intention, plan, select speech means, implement and control speech). These means are personalized depending on what type of statements is "starting" for each child (simple or complex sentence, fragmentary or holistic dialogue, etc.), what are the personal indicators of language capabilities (in terms of diagnostic parameters) and preferences of the child on the subject of statements ("Game," "Animal Care," "Sport," "TV," etc.), what are the personal indicators of each child when performing diagnostic tests (reflected in the appropriate personal diagnostic profile). On this basis, for each child, separate models of statements are selected, objects that motivate the statement, graphic images and problematic communicative situations, individually take into account the variable set of words denoting objects, signs, actions, phenomena; solved range of grammatical and phonetic problems.
Optical-spatial	Means that allow optimizing the training of schoolchildren with SLI and visual impairment, taking into account the peculiarities of the optical-spatial capabilities of these children. These tools provide a linear organization of the stimulus material, its location in space, the possibility of correlating eye movements with hand movements (with tactile and visual row tracking), a fixed increased image size, its contour, detail, etc. These aids are personalized, for example, depending on the recommendations of the ophthalmologist. So children with squint (depending on the squinting eye) are invited to have visual rows on the left (or right); for children with one type of squint, verticalization of images is suggested, and with another type, horizontal position of images. Children in the process of occlusion are given the location of the stimulus material from the "better seeing" eye. Children who are in the process of pleoptic and orthoptic treatment (associated with correcting squint and restoring the ability to fusion-merging two images together) can be offered optical-spatial conditions that are close to those that are suitable for children with myopia (e.g., the increased size of images and their spatial image). The angle of visual stimulus material for children with squint and amblyopia—90 degrees, for children with myopia—40 degrees. When teaching children with myopia, you should monitor the wearing of glasses during class, set a timer that regulates visual loads in time, use "visual pauses" and visual exercises, determine the optimal distance between the eyes of the child and the stimulus material, spatial arrangement of cards relative to each other, etc.

Groups of personalized aids	Characteristics of aids
Light-chrome	Means that take into account the presence of visual impairment in children with SLI. These means provide additional illumination, illumination orientation, and color indication of various actions in the context of holistic activities (e.g., speech-language and subject-practical). These means cause the realization of sufficient illumination of the room, the location of an additional light source for children with squint in the side of the space in which the doctor recommends (e.g., in the state of occlusion), light indicator lights that signal the eye movements horizontally (from left to right) for children with myopia and variably—horizontally or vertically —depending on the type of squint; compliance with the rules of color contrast, the introduction of the contour of the image (e.g., for children with amblyopia—high, medium, or low degree of image contour), its small saturation with small details—for children with myopia and so on. It is necessary to use "anti-glare" materials for graphic presentation—for children with a high degree of amblyopia.
Logical-semantic	Analytical-synthetic tools that help optimize the formation of coherent expressions in children with SLI, taking into account their language and cognitive abilities. These are tools that help analyze, plan, and implement the meaning, content, storyline of statements. These aids are personalized depending on what the indicators of each child are according to the results of the diagnostic profile, what are the difficulties in analyzing and planning speech utterances (difficulties in identifying text composition, transmitting cause-and-effect, temporal, spatial relationships; personal relationships between actors, retelling, creative narration, etc.), what is the nature of difficulties in exercising control over statements (intermediate or final character). Accordingly, for some children it is crucially important to use (as a means) a detailed orated plot analysis, with a consistent analysis of its compositional structure, the introduction of appropriate graphic symbols; for others, it is important to learn to interpret (explain) certain words and expressions, marking difficult to understand and explain words; for the third, strengthening the work on the logic and verbal designation of grammatical relations, and for the fourth, the unification of all these logical and semantic means in the framework of chains and consecutive occupations.
Information technology	Means that with the help of appropriate information technology solutions ensure the formation of coherent statements in SLI children with visual impairment. It can be audio, video, multimedia, telecommunication technology, and so on. Personalization of these funds is determined in accordance with the existing visual impairments, relevant recommendations, and prohibitions from the ophthalmologist.

Table 4.
Personalized aids of forming coherent utterances in children with SLI and visual impairment.

communication). These directions were carried out with the support of conditionally selected groups of personalized teaching aids for children, depending on their content, materialized, technological, visualized, audio, motor saturation.

The identified groups of personalized aids used in the formation of coherent statements in preschool children with SLI with visual impairment are presented in **Table 4**.

The effectiveness of speech therapy work, combining algorithmic, individual, and personalized approaches is much higher than with standard work. These combined approaches are being extremely significant in the light of the accomplishment of tasks to improve the quality of life of children with language impairment and their families.

6. Conclusion

At present, the idea of applying a personalized approach along with algorithmic and individual approaches is very popular and dynamically developing in the context of improving speech therapy in Russia. In particular, aspects of personalized care for children with SLI are being developed. Given the diverse comorbidity of the state of disturbed verbal and nonverbal processes in these children, the personalization of the content, means, and technologies of the speech therapist working with such children will vary significantly, including depending on the scientific, technological, informational, and social resources of society.

The use of a personalized approach in speech therapy seems optimal when there are real conditions for rational integration with other approaches strengthened in science and practice. It depends under competent use of classical and modern scientific data from the field of speech therapy and related sciences, accounting for variable and combinatorial components in the structure of a systemic speech and language impairment understanding of the personalized needs and opportunities of children (social, activity, educational, etc.), the relationship in the work interdisciplinary team of specialists, attracting justified technological solutions, etc.

Author details

Tatiana Volodarovna Tumanova* and Tatiana Borisovna Filicheva
Speech\Language Therapy Department, Moscow Pedagogical State University, Moscow, Russia

*Address all correspondence to: tumanova-t-v@yandex.ru

References

[1] Ushinsky KD. Pedagogical Op. Vol. 6 - T. 2; 1988

[2] Sadovaya VV, Korshunova OV, Nauruzbay Zh. Personalized Education Strategies\\ Mathematics Education. 2016;**11**(1):199-209

[3] Ogarev EI. Specificity of adult institutional education. Human and Education. 2008;**14**(1):64-65

[4] Unt IE. Individualization and Differentiation of Education. Moscow: Pedagogy Publishing House; 1990

[5] Ermakov DS, Osmolovskaya IM, Ryazanova DV. Competency-Based Approach to the Formation of the Content of Education: Monograph. ITIP RAO: Moscow; 2007

[6] Galkina TE. Personalized Approach in the System of Additional Professional Education of Social Sphere Specialists. Avtoreferat of dissertation. D. ped.n.; 2008

[7] Logopedia. Theory and practice. Under ed. Filicheva T. Moscow: Eksmo; 2017

[8] Tumanova T, Filicheva T. Russian scientific trends on specific language impairment in childhood. In: Fernandes FDM, editor. Advances in Speech-language Pathology. Rijeka: IntechOpen; 2017. ISBN: 978-953-51-3510-4, Print ISBN: 978-953-51-3509-8

[9] Levina RE. Pedagogical issues of speech pathology in children. Special School. 1967;**122**(2):121-130

[10] Benilova SY, Davidovich LR, Miklyaeva NV. Speech Therapy Systemic Speech Disorders in Children. Moscow: Sphera; 2014

[11] Specific Language Impairment in Children: Assessment & Intervention Outcomes. Methodical Collection of Materials of the International Symposium of August 23-26, 2018. Publishing House LOGOMAG: Moscow; 2018

[12] Filicheva TB, Chirkina GV, Tumanova TV. The program of speech therapy work to overcome the underdevelopment of speech\language in children. In: Chirkina G, editor. Compensatory Programs for Preschool Educational Institutions for Children with Speech\Language Impairments. Moscow: Education; 2016

[13] Pedagogical Encyclopedic Dictionary. Moscow: Scientific Publishing House "Big Russian Encyclopedia"; 2003

[14] Lalaeva RI, Serebryakova NV. Correction of Underdevelopment of Speech in Preschool Children (the Formation of Vocabulary and Grammatical Structure). Sankt-Petersburg: UNION; 1999

[15] Filicheva TB, Tumanova TV, Eliseenkova OA. Formation of communication of preschool children with a general underdevelopment of speech in gaming activities. Journal Modern Problems of Science and Education. 2014;(3):13-19. http://www.science-education.ru/117-13346

[16] Filicheva TB, Tumanova TV, Gareva TA. The state of speech-lingual processes in preschool children with dysarthria. Journal of Defectology. 2017;(4):22-33

[17] Filicheva TB, Tumanova TV, Guschina YR. Features of word-formation and communicative activity of children of preschool age with speech disorders. Journal Modern Problems of Science and Education. 2014;(6): 21-29. http://www.science-education.ru/117-13346

[18] Filicheva TB, Sokolova TV, Tumanova TV. Formation of coherent utterances in children with primary ocular pathology and specific language impairment. Journal Modern Problems of Science and Education. 2014;(4):74-82. http://www.science-education.ru/117-13346